Public Libraries:
Smart Practices in Personnel

PUBLIC LIBRARIES
Smart Practices in Personnel

PEGGY SULLIVAN
and
WILLIAM PTACEK

LIBRARIES UNLIMITED, INC.
Littleton, Colorado
1982

LIBRARIES UNLIMITED, INC.
P.O. Box 263
Littleton, Colorado 80160

Library of Congress Cataloging in Publication Data

Sullivan, Peggy, 1929-
    Public libraries, smart practices in personnel.

    Includes index.
    1. Public libraries--United States--Administra-
tion. I. Ptacek, William, 1950-   . II. Title.
Z731.S95   027.473   82-15334
ISBN 0-87287-278-5   AACR2

To
Art Murphy
Colleague, Competitor, Friend, and Mentor

TABLE OF CONTENTS

II – PERSONNEL MANAGEMENT AND EVALUATION (cont'd)

III – COMMUNICATION 73

LIST OF ILLUSTRATIONS

Introduction

The nature of personnel practices in public libraries, as in all other institutions, has undergone a good deal of change over the last two decades. At one time, an administrator could hire, fire, transfer, or promote employees on the basis of individual judgment. Now there must be compliance, documentation, and due process. In short, personnel administration has become more involved with legal requirements and contractual agreements. Still, there are many techniques, methods of conduct, and strategies related to personnel work that will greatly benefit public libraries.

Sorting out these smart practices from the maze of required paperwork is not easy. This book is intended to help do that. It is by no means meant to cover all legal aspects of personnel administration. Nor will it cover exactly the requirements for every particular library. Instead, it explains the essentials of personnel administration from the perspective that any public library, regardless of its size or its degree of autonomy from affiliated governments, can develop an effective personnel program. This book focuses on successful strategies for important personnel activities by presenting a logical, commonsense approach to those facets of personnel administration which are most likely to affect public librarians.

The book is divided into three major sections. "Personnel Form and Structure" covers the internal organization of personnel resources, including staffing, position, salary, and benefit structures. It also covers external forces such as budgets, laws, guidelines, and employee organizations that have considerable impact on the overall personnel structure. "Personnel Management and Evaluation" focuses on the day-to-day personnel processes ranging from recruitment to retirement as well as employee relations. "Communication" covers the forms of communication that are crucial to effective personnel administration from such structured activities as collective bargaining, grievances, and interviews, to the more commonplace forms of communication such as memoranda, forms, newsletters, and meetings.

The masculine pronoun is used in this book in its generic sense for reasons of clarity and succinctness. It is intended, of course, to refer to both males and females.

I
Personnel Form and Structure

The form and structure of personnel administration in public libraries evolve from the manner in which the library organizes itself internally and the manner in which it is affected by external forces. In the broadest sense, the organizational structure determines how the work, responsibility, and accountability will be distributed throughout the library. Staffing tables will determine the appropriate size and kind of staff for operational units within the broad structure. Staffing plans require positions that are objectively defined and arranged relative to other positions in the library, and that are in line with similar positions in other organizations. The structuring of positions into a classification scheme forms the basis for a rational compensation program that includes salaries and benefits. The principles and procedures employed by the library to accomplish this structuring should be formally documented in a personnel or staff manual.

Current organizational theory emphasizes that organizations are not discrete, self-contained units. The interaction with outside forces shapes the organization and gives it purpose. This is obviously true of the public library as an institution. The public library responds to the community through the materials it provides and the services it offers. So, too, the personnel practices of the public library are derived from the standards of businesses or affiliated governmental units in the community. These governmental entities may in fact direct the course of personnel administration for some public libraries. City or county governments or local civil service commissions will usually exert the most influence on libraries through the budgeting process. Since personnel and personnel-related expenses make up the greatest part of budgets, this is not surprising. Budgeting for personnel has specific considerations and strategies. On a broader scale, the federal government and state governments, through fair employment practices, regulations, laws, and mandates for employee safety, have a profound impact on the manner in which personnel administration is conducted. Some libraries will be dealing with unions. While these unions will be made up of library staff, they will usually be affiliated with larger organized labor groups and regulated by state laws. Thus, they also produce another important outside influence on the library. Staff associations can play a role in the library's employee relations program. By facilitating communication and adding to the cohesiveness of the library's staff, they may be as beneficial to management as they are to employees.

ORGANIZATIONAL STRUCTURE AND THEORY

The organizational structure of the library is a management tool. In its simplest terms, the structure outlines who does what and who is responsible for what. The structure can help or hinder the operation of the library, but it does not assure either case. There is no best organizational structure. In part, this is because the organization is dynamic. It undergoes constant modification. Management must determine the objectives of the library and then structure the work and relationships in a way that will best accomplish these objectives.

Just as there is no one best organizational structure, there are no hard and fast principles for the development of organizations. However, some concepts are widely accepted. These concepts fit well in most instances of organizational planning. They tend to deal with how the work is grouped and specialized, and how the authority is delegated.

Most organizations, including libraries, are structured so that areas of responsibility with similar objectives are grouped together. Up and down the organizational chart, personnel and operations with similar missions are placed under unified control to take advantage of specific skills and knowledge. This also makes it possible for activities to be easily coordinated to avoid duplication of effort. For instance, branch libraries are grouped together to serve areas away from a central library facility. The abilities of staff and managers in these branches are then combined, and techniques and ideas are shared, so that the limited resources of these branches, in concert with the entire library, can provide good library service to those outlying areas.

In the total picture of a library system, all operations whose purpose is to deliver library service may be grouped under a public services division. Similarly, all operations that are responsible for purchasing, preparing, and processing materials may be combined into a technical services division. Traditional organizational theory holds that this kind of grouping of functions within the hierarchy will yield an efficient library. Likewise, throughout the hierarchy, it is generally thought that the greater the specialization, the more efficient the group will be in attaining specific objectives.

Operations may also be grouped by customers, such as in children's services; by processes, such as maintenance or personnel; and by geographic areas, such as branches, regions, or districts. In looking at divisions of operations, often the terms "staff" and "line" come up. "Line" designates positions that are involved in the actual delivery of services or products. "Staff" designates positions involved in supplying information or services to line units. As the positions take on greater coordinating roles, these terms become less meaningful. Is the director of the library considered part of staff or line? Like most administrators, the director's position includes elements of both kinds of responsibility.

In the analysis of an organizational structure, the concept of span of control is often considered. This involves the number of existing positions and the amount of work that is supervised. There is no magic number of employees that can be effectively supervised. Instead, an effective span of control depends on such factors as the competence of the supervisor, the amount of interaction, and similarity of the units supervised, as well as the extent of standard procedures and unique problems, and the physical dispersion of units.

Perhaps the most crucial guidelines for structuring the organization hinge on authority. Implicit in the span of control and effective grouping is the consideration of how effectively control is maintained. Generally, authority for action should be as close to the scene of action as possible. This delegating of authority or decentralization requires competent management, access to information crucial for decision making, and a situation in which the impact of decisions affects only those units supervised. Only when these conditions are met should authority be decentralized to this level.

The hazard with decentralization is that the authority can become so dispersed that the library becomes too unwieldy for overall management. As mentioned before, there is no perfect span of control. But there is a limit to how much one can supervise. Decentralization "flattens" the organization so that authority for many specifics emanates from the center, leaving too many unit supervisors for top management to control. So there is a limit to the number of positions that can report to one supervisor, but every position must report to only one supervisor. This is a dilemma of organizational planning.

The inherent problem with organizational planning is that two of its fundamental rules of thumb are contradictory. Levels of authority should be minimized through decentralization; yet there is a limit to the number of positions that can be effectively controlled. The best that any library can hope to achieve is a balance between these two principles that will meet the needs of a particular library.

Authority to act always should carry with it accountability. Higher authority is accountable for the actions of subordinates. Classically, authority emanates from the top and filters to the bottom, whereas accountability flows from the bottom to the top. Accountability is tied in with the feedback system that operates up and down the organization. The distribution of authority and accountability and the formal and informal shortcuts make every organization unique. In the end, the organizational structure is the tool of top management that helps the library achieve its greatest potential. The structure creates the environment for a particular style of management. In any work environment, there is a corresponding informal organization. In this informal version, influence, control, and relationships occur with little or no regard to the *legalistic* hierarchy displayed on the organizational chart. (See figure 1 for a diagram of organizational structures.)

Before an existing structure is changed to best reflect the priorities and style of the library's administration, an analysis of the existing structure must sort out the good and bad aspects of the operation. Any subsequent changes should never be motivated by pleasing or by circumventing some people. Organizational change should occur with the understanding that revamping the organizational chart is a most disruptive endeavor, especially when employees feel threatened.

Analysis of the existing structure is the first step. The library director, board of trustees, and the rest of top management should look at their objectives and priorities and compare these with obstacles that hinder their achievement. Such obstacles as conflict within or among units, low level of employee motivation (as evidenced by high absenteeism), overlapping authority, and reduced productivity are good indicators that there is a problem. The trick is to determine if the problem is a result of the structure. For further analysis, management may look at the following indicators: 1) Effectiveness: Are the library's achievements comparable to the library's goals? 2) Flexibility: Can the staff respond well to a changing environment either in the community or in the library? How well did the library or units of the library respond to a crisis? 3) Employee attitudes: While this can be measured by questionnaires, should not an administrator be aware of employee morale? 4) Appropriateness: Does the structure fit the style of

Figure 1. Organizational Structures

TRADITIONAL ORGANIZATION PYRAMID

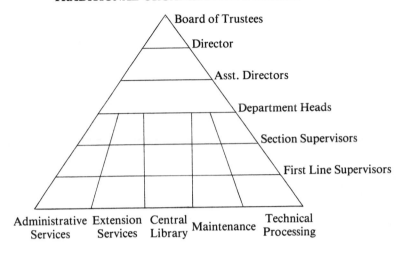

DEPARTMENTAL STRUCTURE

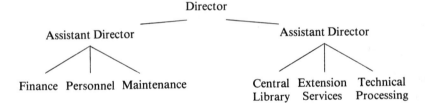

SERVICES STRUCTURE

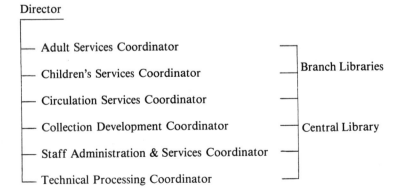

management for the library? 5) Relationships: Can outlining the levels of authority and the span of control on paper make problem areas readily apparent?

If such analysis points to a need to change the organization, the next step is to decide what will be restructured and how this restructuring will take place. The basic organizational structure as outlined by Max Weber is the bureaucratic model that is shaped like a pyramid. In this model, the smallest unit is the director at the top. The number of employees increases as authority is dispersed to the bottom positions. Control is exercised through a chain of command. The variables with this model lie in the grouping of units and their sphere of activities. Although the symmetry may be aesthetically pleasing, the rigidity and over-compartmentalization of such organizations have been longstanding problems.

It is often more fruitful to examine the possibility of organizing units by the processes, groups to be served, or the services offered, and then to decide how these units will be controlled. Special committees or task forces may be created to coordinate the efforts of specialized units. As mentioned before, specialized units may be the most effective way of gaining specific results, but they are also the most costly. While they are concentrating on a project or an aspect of library operation, they may be neglecting or deemphasizing other equally important operations. A library will strengthen itself by having a structure that produces and promotes generalists who, by their knowledge and experience in several aspects of the library's operation, will be better able to facilitate control and aid in the coordination of activities. Specialized groups do not tend to produce such generalists.

Another possible organizational structure includes groups that facilitate control. These internal auditors usually report to top management. They are often in conflict with the middle management that they are bypassing. These groups work within specific time frames to devise strategies or solutions for specific problems. Such groups may be safety committees, committees to improve reference services, and administrative assistants.

Whatever features are included in the new structure, much forethought should be given to avoiding the common hazards of restructuring as identified by Johnston and Woods.* These are:

1. Creation of too many levels of authority
2. Duplication of effort

---

*"Organization and Organizational Planning," in *ASPA Handbook of Personnel and Industrial Relations*, by James I. Johnston and Charles H. Woods, pp. 3-54 – 3-55, Bureau of National Affairs Inc., Washington, DC.

3. Conflicting objectives in the same unit

4. Reporting to more than one boss

5. Improper use of assistants

6. Too many people reporting to a single manager

7. Work loads assigned unevenly

8. Misplacement of functions

The structuring of power in the organization is a related and fascinating aspect of organizational planning. Power may be coercive, associative, expert, or charismatic. In most cases, power will usually develop apart from the way the library is organized. In part, this is because power is conferred by those who are controlled, and in part it is because power depends on the personalities of those who fill the positions. Therefore, it may be wise to pay close attention to who will have access to crucial information. Management will have the right to veto who will represent the library and who acts without permission.

Most libraries do not go through a complete restructuring all at once. When the best structure is decided upon, that structure should become a goal or an objective. Implementing the changes should be as nonthreatening as possible. The earthquake approach is seldom employed. As a general rule, employees need to perceive that the management is competent to administer the changes. They should also be able to recognize the need to change. Changes are usually facilitated by allowing a wide range of participation in the planning stages. Ultimately, if employees see changes in the organization as opportunities rather than as threats to their security, the library is on the right track.

Finally, it should be reemphasized that organizations change without any formal restructuring. Time alone will change attitudes, values, levels of knowledge, experience, and the average age of the staff. A well-managed library will be aware of these changes and will monitor its structure so that it has the best possible environment for the delivery of library services.

STAFFING TABLES

The organizational structure is more fully developed through a system of position control, commonly called a staffing table. All public libraries should develop and use staffing tables. Private sector organizations are not as constrained as public sector organizations by a formal budgeting process. Therefore, private concerns can usually afford to play it loose with the number and kinds of positions devoted to various projects. Public libraries, however, are required to make a public accounting of plans for expenditures. Usually 60-75% of those expenditures involve staff and staff-related costs. For that reason alone, there needs to be a systematic assignment of staff and a rational basis for such assignments. Moreover, library employees are public employees. The public will notice staff that are not actively engaged in some work-related activity. Such negative observations will reflect poorly on the library and ultimately will affect its level of support. Therefore, it behooves the library's administration to make sure that its personnel are properly utilized. Staffing tables serve this purpose and more. They are the library's plan of action for hiring, promotion, reassignment, and budgeting.

Staffing tables designate how many employees and what levels of employees will be allocated to all units of the library. Before these allocations are made, the general organizational structure, down to individual units, will need to be in place, and the specific tasks and responsibilities of each unit must be defined. At that point, consideration of the functions, work load, scheduling, physical size and layout, and other unique requirements for each unit will determine the staffing tables.

The first step is to outline the functions of the unit. A typical branch library, for example, will have reference services, circulation services, and children's services. Collection development, processing of materials, maintenance of the facility, and supervision will also be vital parts of this library. The personnel assigned to that branch library will have to cover all of those functions. Work load in each function is an indication of the quantity of staff needed to accomplish the specific tasks.

In the typical branch library, if the materials are preprocessed, and if materials are selected, and if programs are produced and conducted by another coordinating unit, then the need for staff at that branch may be limited. Circulation counts, number of volumes, number of reference questions received, and number of new volumes added to the collection are all good measures of work load in this case. The complexity of the tasks in each function will dictate the classification level of staff and the degree of specialization required. For instance, a larger staff will require a more competent and experienced supervisor to direct the operation. And if materials are cataloged at that branch library, then personnel with that expertise are necessary. If the circulation system is automated, then the clerical staff must be competent enough to operate the system. On the other hand, if the level of operation is basic enough, the work of the staff may be coordinated so that specific staff members need not be assigned to each function. This is often the case in most public libraries. For example, it often happens that children's services, adult services, and material selection services may be accomplished by one librarian.

Scheduling problems and physical characteristics of the facility are considered next. At the branch library, personnel staff must be available to cover all public service operations during the hours the library is open. Thus, the circulation desk, the reference desk, etc., must be covered during public service hours. Maintenance, however, is not necessarily constrained by the library's public service hours. So the physical characteristics of the facility have other obvious impacts on the staffing requirements. For example, if the branch library is small, personnel may have to carry out many functions from one work station, and maintenance would only require part-time attention.

Every unit will have unique requirements that will need to be taken into account in the staffing tables. Adult and children's services may be so physically separated that two employees are necessary where one would suffice if they were more closely located. The community may be such that security guards need to be on hand. A large facility in a community that is becoming more industrialized may have a diminishing demand and therefore may be staffed by fewer employees than would otherwise be necessary.

When all of these factors are taken into account, a listing of the required staff for that unit may be drawn up. For larger libraries or library systems, allocating staff on a unit-by-unit basis may not be the best approach. If there are a number of similar units (such as branch libraries), it would be more advantageous to compare the measurements of the various considerations mentioned above. Units with similar characteristics can be placed into categories. Staffing tables can then be devised for each category rather than for each unit. Once again, unique factors may require some adjustments across units. Staffing tables, organizational structures, and goals and priorities need constant review. At the very least, the measures that went into devising the plan should be reevaluated to make sure that all units are properly categorized according to those measures or work load.

There are many uses for staffing tables. As mentioned before, they are essential for intelligent budgeting. They provide an organized method for recognizing staffing needs. They are a valuable planning tool, as they can be used to predict the costs of new programs or the cost of shifting existing programs. Staffing tables should include only those positions that are funded. But projected tables, by listing the optimal staffing configurations, can serve as objectives in budget negotiations. Tables listing fewer employees can form the basis of contingent plans in the event of budget cutbacks. (See figure 2 on Developing Staffing Tables for Branch Libraries, page 22.)

Figure 2. Developing Staffing Tables for Branch Libraries

MEASUREMENTS

Branch	Size in Sq. Ft.	Rank	Annual Circulation	Rank	Items in Collection	Rank	Total Rank Points
Argonne	15,500	2	175,000	2	68,000	2	6
Borah	6,000	5	35,000	7	43,000	5	17
Camelot	1,250	9	17,500	9	22,000	9	27
Davidson	10,000	4	100,000	3	58,000	3	10
Ephrem	1,000	10	12,000	10	17,000	10	30
Folger	4,000	6	75,000	6	32,000	6	18
Graceland	2,500	7	90,000	4	26,000	7	18
Henderson	20,000	1	250,000	1	80,000	1	3
Ilchester	1,500	8	20,000	8	24,000	8	24
Joyce	15,000	3	80,000	5	60,000	4	12

STAFFING TABLES

CATEGORY 1 FOR ARGONNE AND HENDERSON BRANCHES
```
 1  Librarian III
 2  Librarian II
 2  Librarian I
 1  Principal clerk
 1  Senior clerk
 2  Junior clerk
 6  Part time clerks
12  F.T.E.* TOTAL STAFF
```

CATEGORY 2 FOR DAVIDSON, BORAH, FOLGER, JOYCE, AND
GRACELAND BRANCHES
```
 1  Librarian II
 2  Librarian I
 1  Senior clerk
 2  Junior clerk
 3  Part time clerks
 9  F.T.E.* TOTAL STAFF
```

CATEGORY 3 FOR ILCHESTER, CAMELOT, AND EPHREM BRANCHES
```
 1  Librarian I
 1  Senior clerk
 2  Junior clerk
 2  Part time clerks
 5  F.T.E.* TOTAL STAFF
```
*F.T.E.: Full time equivalent

EXPLANATION

Branch libraries were ranked according to size, annual circulation, and items in the collections. The cumulated points allowed the library to place the branches into three general categories. Appropriate staffing tables were then developed for each category.

POSITION CLASSIFICATION

Position classification systems for public libraries are most often developed in concert with larger governmental units with which the libraries are associated. These governmental units, such as city or county governments, and frequently civil service commissions, will assist the library with its classification system and subsequently its salary schedules. There are a variety of reasons for this. Primarily, it is to everyone's benefit that all public employees in a given locale are equitably compensated. Moreover, the task of setting up and maintaining classification systems and salary structures is a complex operation that requires a high degree of expertise in personnel administration and industrial relations research. Public libraries do not generally have this kind of expertise in their employ.

From the library's point of view, this cooperative arrangement is advantageous. If wide discrepancies develop in the salary ranges of employees of similar working classes, worker dissatisfaction will follow. Furthermore, if compensation gets out of line with other libraries, employees will leave, and recruiting adequate replacements can become difficult. If such discrepancies exist, employee morale will quickly deteriorate. People do not always need to work under a rational style of management. However, they expect and deserve a rational and equitable system of compensation.

Position classification schemes and salary structures are developed in a well-defined sequence of events. Jobs are analyzed in concrete terms and job descriptions are written. The jobs are then categorized into levels by comparing the relative value of the elements of each job. A hierarchy of positions becomes the classification system. The classes of positions are then compared to positions and salary ranges in similar organizations to determine an appropriate salary schedule.

Job descriptions consist of four basic sections: 1) the job title, 2) the job summary, 3) the listing of duties and responsibilities, 4) the relationships and the requirements of positions. Job titles should be as descriptive as possible and fit into a pattern that is carried out for all positions in the library. It would be inappropriate, for example, to have a series such as Librarian I, Librarian II, and Senior Librarian. The work location should be closely associated with the title (e.g., Librarian II at the Hillside Branch). The job summary is typically a one- or two-sentence definition of the purposes and objectives of the position. The listing of duties, responsibilities, and relationships is the heart of the job description. These may range from a simple listing of the tasks in lower level positions, or they may be narrative accounts of the complex tasks and responsibilities associated with higher-level managerial positions. Requirements for the position include the characteristic skills and the education, experience, and training needed for the position.

There are some universal guidelines for preparing a job description. Although these apply primarily to the listing of duties, they can be used on all parts of the description. Always answer the questions of how, what, who, why. Quantitative terms or descriptions should be used wherever possible. Avoid jargon, as the purpose of the job description is most often to communicate the essence of the position to persons outside the library. It is usually impossible to write an all-inclusive job description. Therefore, the listing of duties, responsibilities, etc. can communicate the essence of these elements by listing illustrative daily, weekly, or annual activities. A crucial aspect of writing good, usable job descriptions is to employ specific and accurate terms that differentiate among the levels of the job. The U.S. Department of Labor has compiled a listing and hierarchy of worker functions, as shown in figure 3. These helpful guidelines should be consulted and used.

Before writing the job description, it is necessary to analyze the job and document its elements. For positions that already exist and are filled, the person in that job can be interviewed or surveyed with an especially designed questionnaire. For new positions, the probable supervisor should provide that information. For public libraries, interviews are usually better than questionnaires as questionnaires are costly measurement tools designed for specific organizations. In any case, the information gathered from either method is categorized into primary functions. For example, the tasks of an adult services reference librarian might be combined into major activities such as reference work, collection development, programming, supervision, and so on.

The first draft of the job description is developed from the categorized listing of activities which are the basis for the summary. The activities within the categories form the listing of duties, etc. The job requirements should be developed by management to conform to prerequisites of similar jobs in similar organizations. All requirements must by law be demonstrably related to the adequate performance of the job. Thus, listing typing skills for a library page whose primary responsibility is to shelve books would be unacceptable. The requirement of a master's degree in library science for professional positions periodically crops up as a controversial issue. Until there is definite proof that this degree is related to future job performance, or until a definite ruling is handed down by the courts, accepting equivalent experience, training, and/or education may be prudent.

The rough draft of the job description should be reviewed by the employee in that position, if there is one, and by the supervisor. When all parties are satisfied with the description, it is good practice to have it

Figure 3. Worker Functions*

DATA	PEOPLE	THINGS
0 Synthesizing	0 Mentoring	0 Setting Up
1 Coordinating	1 Negotiating	1 Precision Working
2 Analyzing	2 Instructing	2 Operating-Controlling
3 Compiling	3 Supervising	3 Driving-Operating
4 Computing	4 Diverting	4 Manipulating
5 Copying	5 Persuading	5 Tending
6 Comparing	6 Speaking-Signaling	6 Feeding-Offbearing
	7 Serving	7 Handling
	8 Taking Instructions — Helping	

DATA

0 Synthesizing: Integrating analyses of data to discover facts and/or develop knowledge concepts or interpretations. Originates, Selects, Edits, Interprets, Designs, Creates, Formulates, Directs, Conducts, Conceives.

1 Coordinating: Determining time, place, and sequence of operations or action to be taken on the basis of analysis of data; executing determination: Plans, Implements, Organizes, Authorizes, Directs, Arranges, Adjusts.

2 Analyzing: Examining and evaluating data. Presenting alternative actions in relation to the evaluation if often involved. Examines, Evaluates, Selects, Reviews, Assays, Studies, Investigates.

3 Compiling: Gathering, collating, or classifying information about data, people, or things. Reporting or carrying out a prescribed action in relation to the information is often involved. Observes, Classifies, Collects, Summarizes, Interviews, Catalogs, Maintains.

4 Computing: Performing arithmetic operations and reporting on and/or carrying out a prescribed action in relation to them. Does not include counting. Calculates, Figures, Quotes, Totals, Determines costs, Makes change.

5 Copying: Transcribing, entering, or posting data. Enters, Records, Transcribes, Posts, Types.

6 Comparing: Judging the readily observable functional, structural, or compositional characteristics of data, people, or things. Sorts, Inspects, Grades, Locates, Verifies, Examines.

(Figure 3 continues on page 26)

*Excerpted from U.S. Department of Labor *Handbook for Analyzing Jobs* (Washington: U.S. Government Printing Office, 1972).

Figure 3. Worker Functions (cont'd)

PEOPLE

0   Mentoring: Dealing with individuals in terms of their total personality in order to advise, counsel, and/or guide them with regard to problems that may be resolved by legal, scientific, clinical, spiritual, and/or other professional principles. Renders, Counsels, Works out, Guides.

1   Negotiating: Exchanging ideas, information, and opinions with others to formulate policies and programs and/or arrive jointly at decisions, conclusions, or solutions. Negotiates, Contacts, Arranges, Participates in talks, Confers, Meets.

2   Instructing: Teaching subject matter to others, or training others through explanation, demonstration, and supervised practice; or making recommendations on the basis of technical disciplines. Trains, Conducts, Provides, Teaches, Coaches, Lectures, Illustrates, Advises.

3   Supervising: Determining or interpreting work procedures for a group of workers, assigning specific duties to them, maintaining harmonious relations among them, and promoting efficiency. Assigns, Has responsibility for, Issues, Directs, Interviews, Establishes.

4   Diverting: Amusing others. Portrays, Performs, Sings, Pilots.

5   Persuading: Influencing others in favor of a product, service, or point of view. Writes, Sells, Promotes, Contacts, Solicits.

6   Speaking-Signaling: Talking with and/or signaling people to convey or exchange information. Includes giving assignments and/or directions to helpers or assistants. Directs, Informs, Indicates, Interviews, Answers, Signals, Receives, Explains, Greets.

7   Serving: Attending to the needs or request of people or animals or the expressed or implicit wishes of people. Immediate response is involved. Receives, Rents, Renders, Carries, Cares for, Stands, Arranges.

8   Taking Instructions-Helping: Attending to the work assignment instructions or orders of supervisor. Helping applies to non-learning helpers.

THINGS

0   Setting Up: Adjusting machines by replacing or altering parts.

1   Precision Working: Using body or tools to accomplish work. Usually involves selection of tools or method.

2   Operating-Controlling: Starting, stopping, controlling, and adjusting equipment.

3   Driving-Operating: Starting, stopping, and controlling the actions of machines which must be guided or steered.

Figure 3. Worker Functions (cont'd)

4 Manipulating: Using body or tools to move, guide or place objects.

5 Tending: Operating equipment with little or no judgement required.

6 Feeding-Offbearing: Inserting, throwing, dumping, or placing materials in or removing them from machines or equipment which are automatic.

7 Handling: Using body, handtools to work, move, or carry objects or materials.

---

formally approved by the library board. Since jobs are constantly evolving because of the various demands placed on employees in their respective positions, it is imperative that job descriptions be updated at least once a year.

Job evaluation is the next step toward the development of salary and classification programs. All positions are placed into a schedule or classification that reflects the relative value of the position. Although there are a number of methods for job evaluation, many are complex and costly evaluation techniques that may be furnished by the encompassing governmental unit. The two principal methods for evaluating jobs are the factor system and the slotting method.

The factor method requires a measurement tool that will be accurate and objective for public libraries, geographic locations, and the kinds of jobs to be evaluated. This tool is a series of factors that apply to the work of the positions in the library, as well as a narrative description of the various levels within the factor (for example, knowledge and training is a factor). The degrees within this factor range from no specific knowledge (requiring only an elementary school education) to highly developed professional skills (requiring a doctoral degree). These, and all degrees in between, are given weighted point spreads. Positions are analyzed by all factors, and a total point value is assigned to the jobs. All positions are then ranked; those with comparable point values are classified into levels.

The slotting method starts by identifying benchmark positions and placing these into a hierarchy of levels. All other positions are reviewed and slotted into levels by comparing them to the benchmark positions.* A reference librarian and file clerk may be benchmark positions at the higher and lower end of the hierarchy respectively. Children's librarian and cataloger may be classed with reference librarian. Junior library clerk and receptionist may be slotted with the file clerk. But while this system may be

---

*This is best done by comparing agreed upon aspects of work such as the amount of supervision or completed work.

adequate for smaller libraries with a smaller mix of positions, a larger library may have several positions that have very different functions and need to be included into a single classification scheme. It would be difficult to pigeonhole an audio-equipment technician, public relations assistant, and marble cleaner into levels that are designed for librarians, library clerks, and children's services specialists. Therefore, larger libraries need a more discriminating technique, usually a factor system, that can accommodate a wide range of jobs.

Here again, job evaluation is an ongoing activity. Whenever all of the positions are reevaluated, there is a substantial cost for implementing all of the changes. Employees' job levels are not reduced because their positions are reclassified. Only when the position is vacant is it placed at a more appropriate lower level. The net effect, then, will be to move current employees into higher levels. Because this is so costly, it is rarely done all at once. A position-by-position reevaluation schedule, spread out over years, is often the best course of action.

SALARY AND WAGE STRUCTURE

Assigning salaries and wages to the classification scheme is another complex operation that, once again, usually requires the aid of the larger governmental unit. Most classification and salary schedules in public libraries fix a value on the position rather than on the individual employee. Each level or grade requires a salary range containing several steps. There is also a prescribed procedure that defines how employees will move up those steps. Rarely will a library have to start a completely new payment plan. Usually salaries are revised to fit the rising cost of living, to keep up with the going rate for similar jobs in the community, or to accommodate a major change in the size and diversity of the library's staff.

Setting salaries is not an exact science. All jobs in the classification schedule must be assigned appropriate salary ranges. The first step is to review current surveys of salaries for key or benchmark positions in each level. Salary surveys for specific geographic locations are available from the Bureau of Labor Statistics, and library-oriented publications often publish salary surveys for professional positions. At this point, a management decision must be made. Will the library adhere to the "going rate" as revealed by the surveys? Does the library's management feel that higher or lower salaries will be adequate to attract and maintain quality personnel? These are decisions that will be based on a variety of factors, including the size of the labor pool in the area, the long- and short-range priorities of the library, and the working conditions the library offers.

Once a change is opted for, be it higher, lower, or the same as the going rate, the salaries in each level are adjusted to a satisfactory level. Classification levels are then plotted against beginning salaries. This usually results in a curve that is either manipulated by mathematics or by inserting additional levels to form a straight line graph. Along this straight line, the difference between grades (levels) is a consistent percentage. Although this straight line proportion is not mandatory, it will insure a rational basis for all levels of salaries that can be easily understood by all employees. Such understanding helps morale.

The steps within a grade are usually consistent percentage increases. The midpoint of the range reflects the salary and experience that the library believes the normal employee should receive when the work is being done satisfactorily. Many salary plans allow for the midpoint to be reached quickly and for subsequent increases to come after a greater length of service. The theory in this case is to promote longevity and reduce turnovers by providing higher salaries for employees with many years of service. This also will distinguish employees with more years of service.

Typically, salary plans call for the beginning employee to be designated as a trainee; he will be raised to the next step after a probation period has been successfully completed. Annual increases, if they are to be merit increases, are granted on the basis of satisfactory performance evaluations. After the midpoint is reached, subsequent increases will occur after 18 months, 3 years, and 5 years of service, respectively. In all grades, the top salary will reflect the maximum amount that the job is worth to the library. At no time should an individual in that grade exceed that amount. If that situation does occur, the library should reclassify the job, or formally move the employee into a position that reflects the salary.

Another salary system involves a series of similar graduated steps within each grade. Increases are based on merit, which is documented at regularly scheduled performance reviews. An exceptional employee may be given a two-step increase; a poor performance may result in only a one-step increase or no increase at all. A prerequisite of this kind of system is that the supervisors conducting the performance reviews are competent enough to be objective and that extraordinary increases will be reviewed by higher authorities.

All jobs should be compared to the standard salary ranges for similar positions in the community. Some positions may be higher or lower than acceptable norms. In those cases, the positions should be regraded to appropriate levels. For example, secretaries may be in high demand in a particular community, which causes the standard salary to be higher than the salary allowed by the library classification. In this case, the library would regrade the secretarial position to a level that would allow for a competitive salary.

If there are many positions that are too high or low, the entire classification system needs to be revised. In some instances, it may be appropriate to offer to start a new employee with special expertise or experience at a higher than beginning step in the grade. This option should be used in rare instances, as employee morale may be adversely affected and the step-in-grade system could be diluted.

The entire salary structure may be adjusted on the basis of a rise in the cost of living. This is a fairly simple task. All steps in all grades are increased by a fixed percentage. Appropriate indications of the shift in the cost of living can be obtained from the Consumer Price Index. Encompassing governmental units will often dictate to libraries what cost of living increases should be granted employees as part of its review of the library's budget request.

The highest administrative positions in the library may be placed in an exempt status. This means that salaries for these positions are based on what the administrator can do, not necessarily on measured output. Salaries are based in large part on the amount the library feels it is willing to pay to have the best administrator it can afford. Here again, comparisons with similar positions in nearby libraries are good indicators of what the amount should be. Using the exempt status classification for the highest administrative positions can also avoid the unwieldy situation where the top manager of the library may be making less money than a subordinate whose longevity has brought him a higher salary. In addition, libraries do not have the same options that private organizations have to offer stock options, bonuses, and other perquisites to top managers. Therefore, it is even more important for libraries to offer competitive salaries in order to attract qualified individuals into their top management positions.

BENEFITS

Benefits can add up to almost one-third of the total personnel costs of the library. As with salaries, norms in the community and the benefit plans of the encompassing government will be the primary determinants of what benefits will be received and how much of the costs of benefits will be covered by the library. Costly mistakes and poor employee relations can occur if benefits are not properly handled, especially when existing benefits are rescinded. Benefits can be a positive factor in recruiting new employees; the absence of benefits can greatly harm recruiting efforts.

There are literally thousands of benefits that can be offered. While it would not be possible to discuss all possibilities, this section will outline the major benefits, illustrate how they can be administered, and point out some important policies and policy decisions for public libraries.

All benefits can be divided into four categories. These are time-off policies, insured benefits, legally required benefits, and special benefits. Time-off policies include sick leaves, vacations, holidays, bereavement leaves, and leaves without pay. All of these leaves require a well-documented and well-publicized policy concerning who qualifies, when they qualify, how much time they can be granted, and how the time off will be approved. Standard practice is to grant time off to permanent full-time and permanent part-time employees (as opposed to temporary, casual, or consulting personnel). The amount of time off within each category is usually based on length of service; some leaves may require a minimum length of service before any time is granted. The actual granting of time off may involve some procedure for notifying the supervisor to allow him time for scheduling and, in some cases, to allow the library board to consider approval. These practices may vary according to the flexibility of the library's managerial style and, more importantly, the library's budget. Time-off policies, while they do not involve direct additional expenditures, can require additional personnel to do the work of those on leave. On the other hand, these costs are partially made up by better morale, fresher, more enthusiastic employees, and a healthier staff. For these reasons, it is impossible to determine the actual cost of time-off benefits.

Sick leave should be granted for well-defined purposes. Some possibilities are illness, health-related appointments, and illness in the immediate family. Sick time is usually earned at specific rates, such as one day per month up to a certain maximum number of days, such as 30 days. Employees who have earned sick leave time, and who must use sick leave, should be given the opportunity to build up their time again at the same rate. Approval for sick leave is a touchy issue. While employees should not always be required to document the cause of the sick leave, the library may want to reserve the privilege of requiring some verification from employees who may be habitually misusing their sick time. There does need to be a procedure for notifying the library when the employee will not be at work (referred to as a call-in procedure). Some organizations offer incentives for employees not to use sick leave. These incentives may be gifts, special recognition, or reimbursement for some or all of the sick time not used at the time of retirement or termination. These incentives can backfire if employees are on the job performing below par or, worse yet, if they are infecting their co-workers.

Vacation is time off with pay. The library's policy should clearly indicate how much time can be allowed for vacation, and how far in advance vacation should be requested. For instance, will the library allow vacation for hours, half-days, or several days at a time? Both of these policies depend on the availability of staff to cover for the vacationing employee. As with sick leave, vacation time is usually earned by the day or in blocks, such as two weeks per year for the first five years, three weeks per year for the next five years, and four weeks per year after ten years of service. Vacation leave is often not allowed until one year of service is completed. It is wise to be cautious about allowing employees to carry over unused vacation into subsequent years. Problems can occur with record keeping and planning. The intent of vacation is to keep employees refreshed by allowing them time to get away and pursue other activities.

Libraries may grant varying amounts of vacation time per year for different employee levels. Professional librarians have customarily been granted four weeks of vacation per year. In order to be competitive in recruiting librarians, it may be necessary to grant four weeks of vacation to those positions, while granting considerably less time to other employees. Benefits can be administered on a different basis for different levels, but they should never be applied differently for individual employees.

Holidays consist of the traditional days such as New Year's Day, Christmas Day, Labor Day, Thanksgiving Day, Memorial Day, Independence Day, and President Day(s). Other holidays may be locally observed days such as Columbus Day, Pioneer Day, etc. Libraries, because they are service organizations, may not close on all locally observed days or on other common days off such as the Friday after Thanksgiving. In order to compensate for this discrepancy with other institutions, the library may want to grant a number of personal holidays each year, which are requested and approved in the same manner as vacation leave.

Bereavement or death-of-a-relative leave should also have well-defined requirements. The most obvious is a definition of what constitutes a relative, which can range from immediate family members to in-laws. The length of this leave should vary with the immediacy of the relative and the time needed to travel to the services.

Leaves without pay are longer periods, usually months or even years, after which the library agrees to bring the employee back at the same or similar position. In some cases the commitment is only to consider reinstatement in the first available opening. The advantage to the library is that it can look forward to the continued service of valuable employees. All decisions concerning the approval of leave or absence must be based on the value the employee has to the library, the length of service, the complexity of the employee's work, and the availability of adequate replacements. Budget constraints must also be taken into account. Can the library afford to go without the employee's service for the time requested? If not, and a replacement is hired, can the library then afford to rehire the employee? Leaves for military service, by federal law, are mandatory and the employee must be rehired at the same level. Leaves for pregnancy must be handled the same as the library's disability leaves. This usually means that the employee is reinstated at the same level when certified as able to return to work. Mandatory leaves for pregnancy are considered discriminatory and therefore not allowable.

Insured benefits represent additional costs to the library. The most prominent of these benefits are life insurance, health insurance, disability insurance, and retirement income plans. More than any other aspect of personnel administration, insured benefits require sound legal and financial assistance. The library must ensure that it does not financially over-commit itself while providing employees and their families with some margin of security in the event of a financially catastrophic occurrence. Expert advice is required to determine if all of these benefits are actually sound. Many insurance plans involve a combination of contributions from the library and from the employees. Rates are often inversely proportional to the number of members enrolled in the plan; it may therefore be beneficial to participate in insurance programs with affiliated government units such as municipal, county, or state employees.

Insurance programs have a wide range of options, deductibles, and coverages. In some cases, it is best to be self-insured. This means that the library will make prearranged payments in the event of death or disability from a prefunded account. The library's plan will depend on what it can afford, how big a group they are associated with, and standard practices in the community. Agents or brokers from the insurance carriers are available to present various plans and options. It is a good practice to have an objective third party broker or a committee of experts advise the library board on insurance matters. For most insured benefits, the insurance carrier, the health maintenance organization, or pension plan group will determine the stipulations of eligibility, waiting periods, and other administrative details. The library has the responsibility to explain the programs in great detail to the employees and to make sure that appropriate deductions are made.

Legally required benefits include federal Social Security, workmen's compensation, and, most recently for public sector employers, unemployment compensation. Social Security laws stipulate that as of January 1, 1981, 13.3% of earned income up to $25,900.00 for each employee be deposited with the Social Security Administration. Half (6.65%) comes from the employee's wages; the other half is contributed by the library. Workmen's compensation is regulated by individual states. In general, the library is liable to compensate employees for pay and medical expenses for accidents, illnesses, or disabilities that are work-related. Depending on the state, workmen's compensation can be covered through a private insurer, a state-controlled fund, or a self-insuring fund. Costs in the first two instances are determined by the number of claims the library submits. The third method, self-insuring, requires that the library has proven assets to cover possible claims. To properly administer workmen's compensation programs, all work-related accidents or illnesses should be reported, documented, and kept on file. In the case of a claim, the insurance carrier or state Workmen's Compensation Agency will need documentation of the incident, of the events and circumstances surrounding the incident, and of the treatment and medical assistance given to the employee as a result of the claim. In addition, a safety program, or at least some attempt to educate employees about possible hazards, may be required for a reduced premium.

Unemployment compensation insurance is state-regulated insurance that will pay an employee a portion (the maximum varies by state) of their wages for 26 weeks after termination. In 1976 this insurance became mandatory for public employees. The cost of this insurance to the library is a sliding percentage of earned income—anywhere from $6,000.00 to $10,000.00. The percentage slides on the basis of the number of claims from the particular institution. Former employees are ineligible for unemployment compensation if they quit voluntarily, if they are discharged for misconduct, if they do not apply for suitable work, or if they are unemployed because they are involved in a labor dispute. To avoid paying claims to ineligible former employees, it is important that the library reply promptly to official inquiries about terminations. For this reason, full documentation of the causes for terminations is absolutely essential.

In addition to deductions for some of the insured benefits, it is customary to make federal and state income tax deductions for all employees on each payroll. Even though federal law requires that only quarterly deposits be made on behalf of employees, the library should make deductions on each payroll to spread out the tax payments. Other payroll deduction plans that the library may want to offer to employees are programs like credit union deposits and contributions to charities such as United Way or Community Chest.

The benefits listed above are but a very few, albeit the most important, of all the possible extras that can be offered to library employees. Other special benefits might include educational assistance, child care, parking privileges, bonuses, transportation, and commercial discounts. Usually these benefits develop through collective bargaining, special abilities of the library to provide such extras, accepted standards for benefits in the particular communities, or through the influence of staff associations. In many cases, public institutions have increased benefits in lieu of salary increases as a way of deferring costs.

STAFF MANUALS

The internal personnel structure of the library is pulled together in the staff manual which basically documents all of the library's policies and procedures that relate to staff and their working conditions, wages and salaries, benefits, and all personnel actions. In addition, the manual can include a description of the organizational structure, the decision-making processes, and the library's goals and objectives.

An updated, well-distributed staff manual is important for a number of reasons. First and foremost, it should be the library's official documentation of policy and procedure. It is the basis for the resolution of disputes, grievances, and even lawsuits. For the management of the library, the staff manual will promote consistency. No matter what changes take place in the administration of the library, the library's policy with regard to personnel issues will be known to all, and subsequent changes will be made public in revisions of the staff manual. The staff will be well aware of the library's policies and procedures concerning such actions as transfers, promotions, salary increases, etc. This should alleviate anxiety and promote a more stable work place.

The staff manual cannot, nor should it, cover all contingencies. Where a formal sequence of events needs to take place, such as with leaves of absence or grievances, the manual should describe the procedure in detail. In other areas, such as public service policies, it will give a general outline that can be adapted to whatever contingencies that arise.

The staff manual must be kept up to date in order to be useful. When staff and time permit, a committee with representatives from the staff, the administration, and the library board can be charged with the ongoing task of updating the manual or, when necessary, completely revising it. In smaller libraries, someone must be made responsible for this task. In all cases, revisions, updates, and additions should be approved by the library board and communicated to the staff.

The American Library Association's Ad Hoc Committee to Revise the ALA Personnel Organization and Procedure Manuals has developed a good outline for staff manuals. The general outline is as follows:*

I. Policies that Affect Employment and Working Conditions

This chapter includes policies of the library and its parent institution that affect or control the services provided by the library and the working conditions of the library staff. Libraries which use

---

*Reprinted with permission of the American Library Association from *The Personnel Manual: An Outline for Libraries.* Copyright © 1977 by The American Library Association.

an Administrative Manual may prefer to publish policies there; in any case, it is important that this information be readily available to all employees.

A. Public Service Policies

B. Affirmative Action Policies

C. State and Federal Fair Employment Practices Laws Applicable to the Library

D. Memorandum of Understanding or Union Contract Applicable to the Library Staff

II. Organization of the Library

This chapter is designed to promote understanding of the working relationships within the library and ways the individual is affected by them.

A. Organization Chart

B. Working Relationships between Units

C. Classification of Positions

D. Process of Implementation and Change

E. Responsibilities of Management and Supervisory Positions

III. Employment Practices

This chapter explains the process by which qualified people are recruited, selected, and appointed to vacant positions.

A. Recruitment

B. Requirements for Employment

C. Selection of a Person to Fill a Vacant Position

D. Appointment

IV. Personnel Actions

This chapter includes all official actions that affect employee's status.

A. Placement and Reassignment within Classification

B. Probation, Performance Evaluations, and Tenure

C. Promotions

D. Resolution of Grievances

E. Remedial or Disciplinary Actions

F. Personnel Records

G. Separation from Service

V. Salary Administration

This chapter explains how each employee's salary is set, the conditions which may affect it, and deductions which will or may be made before the employee receives a paycheck.

A. **Outline of the General Procedure for Determining Salaries**
B. **Salaries and Other Factors Related to Take-Home Pay**
C. **Schedule of Paydays**
D. **Distribution of Paychecks**
E. **Premium Pay**

VI. Employee Benefits

This chapter describes the personal fringe benefits available to employees. Benefits directly related to working conditions are covered in Chapters VII and VIII.

A. **Health Benefits**
B. **Insurance Plans Available, Except Health Insurance**
C. **Retirement Benefits**
D. **Other Fringe Benefits**

VII. Conditions of Work

This chapter includes all policies and regulations which govern the working day. Much of the content may also be in the memorandum of understanding or the union contract, but it is advisable to include all information here, where it can be clearly related to library operations.

A. **Hours of Work**
B. **Special Scheduling**
C. **Overtime**
D. **Disciplinary Action**

VIII. Leaves of Absence

This chapter includes all library or departmental policies and regulations relating to circumstances when absence from work may be authorized. Reference to the memorandum of understanding to the union contract, or to policies of the parent institution (which are included in Chapter I) may be made available either in an introductory section or throughout the chapter. All leave involving "non-pay" status must be clearly identified.

A. **Sick Leave**
B. **Maternity Leave**

C. **Vacation**
D. **Holidays**
E. **Personal Leave or Floating Holidays**
F. **Compassionate or Funeral Leave**
G. **Leave without Pay**
H. **Attendance at Conference, Meetings, Workshops**
I. **Sabbatical Leave**
J. **Industrial or Occupational Sick Leave**
K. **Other Leaves of Absence**

ASSOCIATION WITH OTHER GOVERNMENTAL UNITS

Public libraries have varying degrees of autonomy in relation to local governments, ranging from totally independent library districts to libraries that are departments of local government. The most common situation is for the public library to be governed by its own policy board, while budgets are appropriated through the local government, such as a city council or county commissioners. Aside from these formal ties, there may be different levels of interaction between the library and local government administrations. Tax revenues may be certified through the governmental units; otherwise the library may be a totally independent operation. In some cases, all expenditures may be required to be processed and approved through the offices of the local government, and a centralized personnel office may direct the library's personnel administration.

Since the beginning of the public library movement in this country, public libraries have generally been recognized as institutions of common benefit to the community. Libraries often sprang up as a result of local effort, including a good bit of volunteer effort and philanthropy. Sometime later, the responsibility for maintaining and continuing the development of the libraries was given to local governments. However, for many reasons, including the unique educational role of libraries and the undesirability of undue political or religious influence on the choice of materials and services in the libraries, independent policy boards were usually charged with the responsibility of directing the library.

This somewhat contradictory relationship, in which the library is responsible to the local government and yet is controlled by an independent board, has often led to poor relations between the library and the associated governments. Library administrators in this situation often perceive an ongoing struggle to maintain autonomy. The biggest problem is that financial support from local government may require giving up some discretion. This issue crops up frequently in the area of personnel administration.

Personnel administration in the public sector has had an interesting, though somewhat tainted, history. The United States has had a tradition of electing many more public officials to more levels of government than other countries. A natural outcome of this is the common practice of employing public employees on the basis of political considerations. Hence, the spoils system and patronage system developed quickly; in some communities they are still in existence.

Between 1880 and the early 1900s, public disapproval of these practices led to civil service reform, resulting in laws designed to ensure that government workers were hired on the basis of abilities and competence rather than on the basis of whom they knew or supported. Over the years, civil service has become cumbersome and, in some cases, counter-productive. The rigid classification systems and salary schedules based on seniority gave public employees little incentive to go beyond the minimum requirements of their jobs. Lists of eligible candidates for civil service positions severely limited recruitment. The cumbersome bureaucracy for handling personnel actions such as promotions, reclassifications, and terminations severely limited the flexibility and discretion of public administrators to manage personnel.

More recently, the enactment of affirmative action laws, the increased public demand for efficiency, and better cost control in government functions have caused the public sector to move away from civil service. In its place, competent professional personnel offices and competent managers have developed. Because the public sector is generally subject to the same regulations as the private sector, and because of the growth of public employee unions, there is often little difference between the private and public sector personnel management.

It is no wonder, then, that there should be some concern for autonomy, given public libraries' history of development apart from other public agencies, the libraries' unique status of being a part of local government with separate governing bodies, and the history of public employment tainted with patronage and inefficiency.

However, as personnel administration becomes more expensive and complex, as public sector personnel administration becomes more professional and competent, and as libraries need more support, the prospect of working with local government becomes more attractive. By joining with larger public agencies, the library can reduce costs for many benefits such as health and life insurance and retirement income programs. The expertise and resources of local governments' centralized personnel offices can assist the library in developing classification and salary plans that they could never afford to develop on their own. Likewise, recruitment in the form of referrals, and advertising through a larger pool of applicants can also help in reducing costs and in finding better employees. The price to pay for these and other benefits is often the loss of some autonomy. The library administration must determine what is best for the library and foster the encompassing governmental units in such a way that the price does not become too high.

BUDGETING FOR PERSONNEL

Budgeting is a most crucial aspect of library administration. The budgeting process consists of preparing, presenting, and gaining approval of the library's budget. Although budgets are annual, the process is usually very time-consuming, as the budget request must filter down through several levels of authority—including the library board, the review officials, and a legislative body. This process requires the library administration to be adept at planning, accounting, and politicking, as it will be competing with other departments for limited funds and will be getting pressure from the public to keep costs down. Because personnel costs can amount to from two-thirds to three-fourths of the library's budget, personnel considerations are a predominant factor in the budgeting process.

Library budgets are developed through one of three methods. Line-item budgeting is the oldest and still the most utilized method of budgeting, using categories of expenditures from the previous year. Planned-program budgeting categorizes expenditures into programs and compares these expenditures with measures of productivity to arrive at cost-benefit ratios. Zero-based budgets isolate functions of the organization, dividing them into levels of activity with the corresponding cost and results. These budget methods are called decision packages. Whatever method is used, the basic principles of budgeting remain the same—What do you want to do? How much will if cost? How little can you get by with? How will you convince the powers that be to grant your request?

The first step in determining personnel budgets is to look at next year's programs and functions and determine how many more or fewer staff will be needed, and what level of staff will be needed to carry them out. All projections of future personnel costs will need to take into account the following items: pay increases, including across-the-board cost-of-living increases; merit or longevity raises for individual employees; salary increases due to promotions, increases from union contracts; and the corresponding adjustments for benefits usually based on salaries. It is important to remember that in setting up personnel budgets the library is developing or maintaining budgeted positions within the framework of some overall plan through staffing tables or some organizational staffing plan. This way personnel can always be tied back to specific programs and services.

Justifying budget requests is at the heart of the budgetary process. It is usually not enough to demonstrate that a program is deserving. The decision makers, be they elected officials, legislators, a budget review staff, or the public, must be convinced that they are getting the best value for their money. Unless the library takes that stance, there is little chance that library programs will be compared favorably to programs such as police and fire protection. Demonstrating the value of money spent on library programs requires strategies that are designed to fit particular situations. There are as many strategies as there are administrators who must submit budgets.

Budget requests are almost always reduced as they move through levels of approval. Therefore, it is smart to start high and know the critical point at which the reduction is too drastic. In terms of personnel, this means justifying staff increases by showing need and results. Higher circulation, more materials to process, more demand for reference assistance, expanded hours of services, and more facilities are but a few such possibilities. The important point of this strategy is to tie staff increases to concrete programs and demonstrable results. Often, comparisons with other libraries can accomplish the same thing. Meeting the standards developed from the results of a planning process system can be helpful. ALA's *A Planning Process for Public Libraries* (American Library Association, 1980) can be a useful tool to develop such goals and standards.

Because budget approval is a form of negotiation, the library must know what programs are negotiable. Unless there are severe limitations on available revenues, budget authorities are reluctant to reduce the existing work force. The library can show good economizing effort by reducing staff positions for programs that may be expendable and transferring these positions to more promising or worthwhile activities. For example, the staff from a discontinued bookmobile service can be transferred to a new branch library. That way the library starts a new program, the community officials show an economic cutback, and the employees remain employed.

Another productive strategy is the "foot-in-the-door" approach. In this case, the library would request the bare minimum to begin a new program, anticipating that future budgets for the project will be increased. This usually works best with line-item budgeting because it lends itself to using last year's budget as a base for increases in subsequent years. Here again the program must be popular, as proven by measurable results.

The best overall strategy for budgeting is to prove the library's worth all year long. It is a difficult proposition to convince local officials to support the library and its programs if they have not had good feedback about the library. That is why an organized approach to managing personnel resources is integral to successful budgeting.

FAIR EMPLOYMENT PRACTICES

Federal regulations pertaining to fair employment practices have entirely changed personnel practices and procedures. Federal laws have been aimed at the elimination of discrimination because of age, sex, or race in recruiting, hiring, and all other manner of personnel administration. These changes are the result of the Civil Rights Act of 1866 and 1877, Title VII of the Civil Rights Act of 1964 (and its amendment of 1972), and the Equal Pay Act of 1974, to name a few. More recent legislation has expanded coverage of most of these laws to cover public, hence public library, personnel practices.

The cornerstone of compliance with this often confusing body of regulations is an affirmative action program. While many public libraries may not be obligated to have an affirmative action program, they are required to file EEO-4 reports to the Equal Employment Opportunity Commission directly or through their encompassing governmental unit. Libraries with over 100 employees must file an annual EEO-4 report that details its affirmative action progress and plan. Libraries with 15 or more employees are required to compile information used in this report and be able to file it upon request. More importantly, the libraries must comply with most of the regulations that private sector organizations comply with so that it makes sense to organize the effort into an affirmative action plan.

The basic elements of an affirmative action plan are the following:

1. A statement of the library's commitment to equal employment opportunity and to personnel actions which will be taken without regard to age, race, nationality, sex, religion, or handicapped status in cases *where these may be bona fide qualifications for a job.*

2. An assignment of responsibility that stipulates the library's agent responsible for the implementation of the plan.

3. A policy on communicating the plan to the employees and the public.

4. A utilization analysis that lists the various job groups, identifies the protected individuals (minorities) in those groups, analyzes the availability of protected individuals for the job groups in the community, and a comparison between

the ratio of protected individual employees and the availability of protected individuals in the community.

5. The goals and timetables for correcting deficiencies in job groups.

6. Indication of problem areas where selection criteria have had an adverse impact (defined by a selection rate of less than four-fifths minorities to nonminorities).

7. A system for reviewing progress or developments of the program with supervisory personnel and for reviewing statistics or mandatory reports.

Affirmative action implies that the library will not only hire qualified protected status individuals when they apply for actual job openings, but that the library will actively recruit such minorities to fill positions in job groups that have too few minorities. Recruitment itself must be nondiscriminatory in its content and method. Job announcements should in no way indicate discrimination. All requirements for vacant positions must be job-related, which is defined as having a statistically significant correlation to the performance of the job. If the requirements (proficiency tests, educational attainment, etc.) yield an adverse impact on the selection of protected status applicants, the library may be forced to validate the requirement to show that it is job-related. Jobs must be advertised in such a way that all segments of the available pool of protected classes have an adequate chance to find out about them. Referrals, word-of-mouth advertising, and any other informal methods of recruitment are not acceptable if they systematically exclude minorities from applying.

Before hiring an individual, the library should refrain from inquiring about race, marital status, national origin, religion, and any other personal information that could be construed as discriminatory. This applies to employment application, screening interviews, and any personal contact with the applicant before hiring. Pre-employment inquiries about race, sex, or national origin are permissible if they are asked for the purpose of gathering data for EEO-4 reports. This is usually done with a rider, attached to the application form, which does not identify the individual by name. Just as the formal requirements for a job cannot be discriminatory, the actual criteria used to select a candidate must be job-related or they will be considered unfair. Criteria such as sex, age, national origin, religion, co-worker preferences, and marital status can rarely be proven to be job-related. Criteria of educational attainment, experience, and physical and mental aptitude are fairly safe as long as they relate to appropriate jobs and do not systematically exclude protected status individuals from those job groups.

Similar nondiscrimination regulations apply to the employees of the library. The assignment of work, the use of facilities, the levels of compensation, and the dress requirements must be uniformly administered. Benefits, such as leaves of absence, insurance coverage, and other privileges, cannot be held back for protected classes of employees. Opportunities for training, transfer, or promotion must be equally accessible to all qualified employees. The library should also be careful to document all disciplinary actions so that they can be proven to be non-discriminatory. These are but a few of the regulations pertaining to fair employment practices. The Commerce Clearing House *Guidebook to Fair Employment Practices, 1979* (Commerce, 1979) is a very readable summary of all pertinent regulations. Since the laws in this area are still evolving, it is important to be aware of the latest rulings, amendments, and new legislation on both the state and federal levels.

Libraries with over 100 employees must file an annual EEO-4 report that details affirmative action progress and plans. Libraries with 15 or more employees are required to compile information used in this report and be able to file it upon request.

SAFETY

The safety of employees has considerable legal and financial implications for the library. In 1970, the Occupational Safety and Health Act (OSHA) made it mandatory for private organizations to conform to a set of standards for employee and work place safety and to rectify any recognized hazards in the plant or facility. OSHA does not apply to state and local public employees unless the particular state has passed legislation for public institutions. However, all libraries need to be concerned about safety. First, there is the humanitarian concern that employees be provided with a hazard-free environment in which to work. Another consideration is the costs involved with work-related employee accidents and illnesses. Workmen's compensation rates are directly tied to the number of claims that have been received from the library. Also, property damage to the library facility in the event of a catastrophic incident will be costly. The key elements of a safety program are preventing incidents through training, increasing safety awareness, and reviewing and planning for emergency situations.

A good program of accident prevention will first identify problem areas and activities. Insurance carriers can be called upon to inspect the library facility and work procedures to identify the problems before they result in personal or property damage. Other sources of help for such reviews are local building, electrical, and fire inspectors. Where hazards in the facility, equipment, or tasks have been identified, alternatives should be worked out. If the situation cannot be altered, employees should be made aware of the dangers and be trained in safe procedures to avoid accidents.

The most critical aspect of prevention is employee awareness. This awareness can be generated through staff meetings, training programs, or notices and written communications to employees. When the size of the library warrants it, a safety committee should be responsible for awareness campaigns. If a committee is not feasible, at least one staff member or administrator should be responsible for safety in the library.

Notwithstanding prevention, it is inevitable that work-related accidents will occur. It is imperative that a mechanism be in place to handle such incidents. Report forms should be on hand to document the accident. Injured employees should be referred to a particular doctor and health care facility. All staff should be aware of these arrangements. Staff should also have at least some rudimentary training in first aid and cardiopulmonary resuscitation if possible.

The best way to handle a future emergency such as fire, bomb threat, power failure, or robbery is to have a plan for the emergency and have the staff review and practice the procedures that have been set up. For example, preparing for fires would mean that each staff member be assigned a method of exiting the building. Also, there should be a plan for clearing the building of patrons during public service hours. Most importantly, fire drills should be held throughout the year at various times of the day and on different days of the week.

UNIONS

The growth of unions in the public sector has been so dramatic in the last two decades that unionized public employees now exceed the number of unionized employees in private industry. Public libraries have not been immune from this organizing effort. Typically, employees of similar vocational interests, such as those in professional, clerical, or maintenance positions, form bargaining units that serve as the sole bargaining agents for those classes of employees with the library administration. A true union situation does not exist unless the union has the right and responsibility to meet and confer with or bargain with the library administration for terms and conditions of employment.

Unions become exclusive bargaining agents after a petition is signed by the state-specified percentage of the affected employees. The petition mandates an election in which a majority vote in favor will give the union exclusive bargaining rights. Of course the library administration must still recognize the union and agree to negotiate the terms and conditions of employment. Unlike the private sector where a number of federal laws make the whole process rather cut and dry, and where the National Labor Relations Board is available to settle any disputes, the public sector is guided by state and local laws that are in no way uniform or consistent.

Recognizing unions and negotiating contracts with public employees have had a tumultuous history. Public officials have been reluctant to deal with organized labor unions for a variety of reasons. The most frequent argument against public employee unions has been the conflicting principles of the political sovereignty of the institution and the right of public employees to bargain collectively. Unlike private industry, libraries are governed by trustees who ultimately must answer to a higher authority, the electorate. Options for funding, relocation, or even continuing the existence of the library are not at the discretion of the library's administration as they would be in private industry. By agreeing to negotiate terms and conditions of employment, public officials may be giving up their decision-making powers to a negotiator, or even a mediator, if some sort of arbitration is employed to settle contract disputes. However, this argument was considerably diminished in 1962 when President Kennedy signed Executive Order 10988, which gave federal employees the right to organization and to collective bargaining. Since then, most states have recognized the rights of public employees to organize some form of unions.

Despite the emergence of state and local legislation protecting public employees' right to organize, the library administration may want to discourage unionization for a variety of reasons. Management's first and foremost consideration is to avoid any job actions by any bargaining units. Strikes, work stoppages, or slowdowns will not help to promote the library. Even if local laws do not permit such actions, it has been demonstrated across the country that public employee unions can and will make use of their primary method of influence—the strike.

Further concerns about unionization focus on the inflexibility and conflict it can impose on personnel relations. A union contract may severely limit the library administration's ability to allocate resources or to take disciplinary action without getting involved in a sometimes lengthy grievance procedure. Unions may affect the professional status of librarians who may be so entwined with management or supervisory functions that unionization would exclude professionals from bargaining units. If they are included, it places professionals in an uncomfortable middle ground where they must be responsive to employee rights as well as management decision making.

At this stage in the evolution of public sector collective bargaining, there may be even greater negative aspects to unionization created by the effect of outside factors. Many successful union efforts in public libraries have relied on affiliation with larger unions such as the AFL-CIO-affiliated AFSCME. It is possible that outside professional negotiators may be called in to bargain for the employees who have little feeling for the political or economic constraints on the library. For example, the effect of a successful property tax initiative will certainly impinge on the library's ability to grant significantly higher wages. There is no guarantee that the union will be responsive to the constraints on a public institution. Furthermore, public sector collective bargaining is by no means adequately regulated in every state. There is no uniformity in many states' approaches to several key aspects of public employee unions and collective bargaining. Such aspects include the right to strike, contract mediation in lieu of the right to strike, the responsibility to recognize and bargain with legitimate unions, the conflict between union contracts and local civil service laws, and unfair labor practices. In short, this country has no uniform legislation to provide for the orderly conduct of labor relations in the public sector as it has for the private sector.

In the event that the library decides to counter a unionizing effort, there are several useful measures that can be taken. Management should first of all be aware of all potential or actual attempts to unionize. There should be an effective employee relations program that keeps the library in touch with employees' concerns and that can communicate some of the uncertain or negative aspects of a union for the employees. Most importantly, an adequate compensation program will help alleviate employee dissatisfaction, the most frequent cause of unionization. In any of these measures the library must be careful to avoid infringing on the employees' right to organize. Such infringement could be ruled as an unfair labor practice.

There are positive aspects to unions in the library. Collective bargaining can be an organized method for achieving good employee relations. For employees, collective bargaining can bring better compensation, more evenhanded treatment, and a greater role in determining work environment. For management, collective bargaining can result in better communication with employees, formalized personnel policies, and an enhanced status for management personnel. The key element for a mutually beneficial labor relations situation is awareness. Management and employees should be aware of each other's concern and constraints, and this awareness should be translated into reasonable positions in all aspects of labor relations.

STAFF ASSOCIATIONS

Although staff associations do not have the legal force of recognized unions, they often play an important part in the relationship between library employees and administration. A good staff association will facilitate communication. It can channel employee interests and concerns informally to management on one hand; on the other hand, the staff association can act as an acceptable mechanism for management to respond to employees and to consult with them about policies, ideas, and plans. In other areas of employee relations, staff associations can assist with continuing education, social functions, and additional employee benefits.

A staff association should be independent of the library's administration. Its strength should come from the support of the staff. Management should not attempt to co-opt the staff association so that the association will maintain credibility and so that management can look to this group for truthful, meaningful dialogue.

Aside from its role as facilitator for communication with management, the staff association can be an effective conduit for information among staff members. This frequently is done through newsletters and meetings. However, staff-association-sponsored lectures, workshops, and symposia can be a valuable source of work-related information for all employees. For instance, such presentations could focus on procedures, issues, or operations pertinent to the particular library, like civil service regulations or a revised staff manual. Moreover, they could inform the staff about relevant developments outside of the library that may affect them in the future, like automated circulation systems or library legislation.

The social value of an active staff association should not be overlooked. Staff-association-sponsored social events can be catalysts for better morale. When employees become more aware of one another and their work, the cohesiveness of the library staff will be enhanced. This is true even in small libraries. This kind of organization can also assist employees in obtaining additional fringe benefits, ranging from better rates for insurance to reduced costs for purchases from local businesses or discounts for recreational activities. In any case, the library administration should support and foster staff association efforts without attempting to direct or control them.

II
Personnel Management and Evaluation

Throughout the association of any employee with the public library, there is a series of processes that involve initiatives by the library and responses and initiatives on the part of the employee. The ways in which these are orchestrated can be done well, and when they are, job satisfaction, staff morale, and the positive realization of the library's goals are enhanced. These processes include recruitment, appointment, transfer, promotion, leave of absence/reinstatement, retirement, resignation, termination, training, staff development, and employee counseling. These processes, and related record keeping to make the processes occur in an efficient and timely manner, are treated in this section.

RECRUITMENT

Even when there are not many opportunities for employment of additional staff, recruitment is a significant part of the personnel function. Perhaps more than some of those functions, it needs to be well understood by the staff as a whole, and it can benefit from the continual assistance of the staff as well as other members of the library's community who may aggressively seek the best staff for appointment or be informed of the status of personnel needs so they can respond intelligently to requests they may receive about library employment.

Although opportunities to employ may occur sporadically and with short notice, the recruitment process makes it possible to maintain a pool of candidates for positions from which selections can be made. Systematic advertising of positions assists in this process. Especially in beginning-level positions, there may be an advantage to the library in announcing the types of positions available on a seasonal basis. For example, at the time June graduates from high schools or community colleges are seeking work, posting information about the kinds of positions available may call the library to the attention of graduates whether or not they are at that time interested in such opportunities. The administrator responsible for personnel must determine, after some experience with advertising, whether it is worthwhile to recruit in this manner by assessing the qualifications of persons attracted to the library, jobs available, and the time required to consider those who come.

Some of these same concerns apply when deciding the ways to advertise librarians' positions. In times when the number of library school graduates may exceed the number of openings available, some administrators fear being flooded with inquiries and applications that complicate, rather than assist, their task of recruitment and selection of librarians. As with the announcement of positions to high schools and colleges, some selection may need to be made among the institutions approached. When doing this, the administrator should consider the present composition of the staff, deciding whether some institutions have provided good recruits in the past, but also allowing for the desirable diversity of educational background that can improve the quality of staff. For example, while one nearby institution may offer a library education program that has produced most of the library's staff members in the past, there may be value in adding to the list of those to which information about job opportunities is mailed institutions which may, according to their mission, be preparing students in the skills and attitudes most needed by the library at a given time. Similarity of goals may be more significant than such characteristics as geographic location, size of classes, or aggressiveness of placement activities on the part of the educational institutions.

Many recruits to library positions may come from the less easily identified pools of those returning to employment after a period of family responsibilities, those seeking changes of employment, and those new to the library's community. Formal and informal means of communication are needed to attract and inform these prospective employees. Among the informal means, an important channel is the library staff. Individual staff members may receive inquiries in the course of their work from people who think they wish to do similar work, or they may encounter people in social settings who ask about the possibility of employment. In some instances, staff members may be impressed with the skills and interests of individuals whom they wish to recruit to the staff. Whatever the source of the interest, it is important that all staff members be familiar enough with the process of employment that they can refer individuals directly to the office or the individual who can provide the information the prospective employee needs about how to apply for a position. There is nothing more frustrating to a would-be staff member than to be referred and re-referred to several people when seeking the information that may lead to employment. When the person is anxious to seek employment, poor referral can add to anxiety, and, perhaps more significant to the library, good prospective employees can be lost to the institution because they are frustrated by their initial encounters with it.

Advertising in library periodicals is frequently desirable. For some higher-level positions, nationwide recruitment efforts may considerably enhance the pool of candidates and may be required for affirmative action compliance. Careful consideration should be given to which journals are used, with frequency of publication, time requirements for deadlines, target audience within the library profession, and costs of announcement taken into account. The political entity within which the public library functions may also have access to journals in which some positions should be posted. Familiar as library administrators typically are with the standard journals of librarianship, they may need to review the possibilities for placing announcements in the journals of other fields when they are recruiting people in supervisory or administrative posts in such specialties as data processing, supervision of custodial or maintenance personnel, or finance.

Joblines, electronically recorded announcements of positions available, are maintained by some state libraries and some library organizations. Public libraries should consider using those that are likely, because of geographic location, to produce applicants for positions to be filled.

Newspaper advertising naturally reaches a broader readership than library journals. Local newspapers may be the major means of stimulating applications for clerical positions in the library, and they may also be useful in announcing professional positions. Better targeting of announcements may occur when newspapers can provide sections for the announcements of library positions, and these sections are a good device to call to the attention of a wide public the range of opportunities available in librarianship. Major newspapers, such as *The New York Times* and *The Chicago Tribune*, should be considered for advertisements even by libraries outside their immediate geographical areas.

The preparation of advertisements is worth the time and thought necessary to make them clear, honest, and forceful. Terseness is usually desirable for reasons of economy, but heavy reliance on abbreviations is usually an indicator of poor communication rather than of thoughtful economy. The first words of the printed advertisement should indicate the specialization required in the position. If children's librarians, reference assistants, and bookmobile librarians are all needed by the same library at the same time, separate announcements directed to people in those specializations should be prepared. Catch-all ads do just that: they catch all, rather than catch the potential staff members desired. The administrator should also be aware of the fact that the library profession is relatively small, and individuals may look askance at a library that regularly announces job openings or that repeats the job announcements. Mention of opportunities made possible by new bond issues or increased scope of the library or reference to promotional opportunities that have opened up lower-level positions may be additional impetus for people to follow up on the advertisement.

Once possible applicants have been identified by the library, the process of selection begins. Every inquirer or applicant deserves the courtesy of a reply to the inquiry or application. Simple notices of receipt of applications should be sent. Applicants whose backgrounds suggest they are the most likely candidates should receive information about the interviewing process, the possible date by which selection will be made, and further details about the position. If a specific application form needs to be completed by persons interested in positions, it should be available in sufficient quantity that it can be sent in a routine fashion to those who have indicated an interest in applying for positions. The application form itself should require the applicant to give sufficient information to make it easy to record the application, communicate with the applicant, and have sufficient information about previous work experience, educational background, and references so that the application, when read by individual staff members in the library who are participating in the selection process, will present as complete a picture of the applicant as possible.

It is desirable for applications to be logged and recorded so that action on them can be reviewed as necessary. The administrator responsible for personnel management may have the file maintained in one location, but applications that are being considered most seriously should be available to the supervisors who may be responsible for the selection of individuals for employment. It is useful to have the less likely applications weeded out at an early stage, but they, too, should be available in case questions arise about selection or in case individual staff members participating in the selection process ask to see them to verify the initial decision.

Good personnel practice includes retaining applications and, to the extent possible, reviewing them periodically to see whether persons who applied for one position might be approached either to apply for or to be interviewed for another position if they were not chosen for the one in which they were originally interested. Such files are difficult to maintain and, in most instances, the memory of the person responsible for personnel is a valuable asset in retrieving such information from the application files.

Periodic review of the application files is also a good means to evaluate the processes of advertising and announcing positions. If the ratio of unlikely applications is higher than should be expected, it may be that faulty or insufficient information was included in the announcement of a given position.

It is desirable, but not essential, to have more than one applicant available for consideration by interview. The most costly part of interviewing is the investment of time on the part of the staff participating, so that investment should be carefully organized and monitored. The interviewee's time is also valuable, and the interviewee's schedule may be difficult to arrange if the interview is being scheduled within a busy schedule of work or school. In most instances, the library is not expected to pay the cost of travel or accommodations for the person being interviewed, but, obviously, in instances where the library is attempting to attract an individual for a high-level position, or where the reputation and application of the individual suggest the need to be aggressive in recruitment, the offering of paid expenses may be a useful incentive.

Group interviews are sometimes a good device to get the opinion of several staff members in a limited period of time. These also make it possible for individual staff members to observe different means of communication, listening skills, and body language of the applicant. In these instances, it should be clearly understood before the individual applicant is interviewed, what the ground rules are: how long the interview should be, what the pattern of questions will be, and how the individual interviewers will assess and merge their own evaluations.

The purpose of interviewing is twofold: the potential employer has an opportunity to ask more specific information about the applicant's skills, interests, and potentials with regard to the specific job available, and the applicant can find out details of the job and information about the institution that might not have been readily available before. The interview should be thorough and should occur after the provision and the careful perusal of all written material that may help either part of the process, the applicant or the employer, to determine the individual's appropriateness for the position.

Throughout this process, both the individual and the library have rights and responsibilities. Applications may need to be reviewed by several people, but they should be treated as confidential. Commitment to an interview should indicate on both parts an openness to the decision about the position. Time is too valuable to be spent on nonproductive interviews, and, if the library is not going to employ the individual based on information already available, it is not fair to require the individual to come for an interview. On the other hand, the applicant who has already made a commitment to another position or who, for any reason, does not intend to accept the position if offered it should withdraw before being interviewed.

At the time of the interview, it may be desirable for the library administrator to give the applicant some idea of the time-line for decisions about employment. Estimates of how long it may take until applications and interviews are completed, how long after that it might be until the appointment could be confirmed and the successful applicant begin work, and similar details are useful to know. Too often, the interviewer, in an attempt to be encouraging, leaves the applicant with the impression that there are only some formalities or approvals to be obtained, when the facts needed to make a decision are not yet all available. At the time of the interview, any other requirements relating to application and employment should also be verified, such as residence requirements, necessity to participate in pension plans, permission to communicate with references or with present employer.

Concerning the references that an applicant provides, there are several different patterns of practice. Sometimes the applicant may be asked to provide the potential employer with the names and addresses of people who can comment on the individual's academic and/or work experience, personal characteristics, etc. The employer may then write or telephone them to request information about the individual. Sometimes this communication is not pursued until after the interview, at which time it may be useful for the interviewer to ask the applicant why these references were chosen and the special knowledge or information they may have to offer about the applicant's background. If the applicant's present supervisor or employer is not included in this group, the potential employer may wish to ask for permission to communicate with this person, but it should be understood that this communication might be awkward if the applicant has not informed the present employer of interest in changing positions. The applicant should be allowed some lead time to inform the present employer or supervisor that an inquiry may be coming from the potential employer.

In some instances, the employing library may follow the practice of asking applicants to write directly to possible references and to have them communicate with the library. If any specific information, such as length of time the reference has known the applicant, is required, the applicant should be informed of it so that it can be requested.

When a specific number of references are required, it should be understood that there might be extenuating circumstances that could prevent one or two of the references from replying at a given time. If it is essential to have a certain number, the applicant should be informed if any have not answered within a reasonable period of time and allowed to ask for substitutions. Travel, illness, or change of address are only a few of the reasons why one or more persons might not respond as promptly as hoped.

Some educational institutions maintain placement files for their former students or alumni. These may include references acquired over a period of years as well as those written during or soon after the individual's student days. While review of these files may be useful for the library considering the individual for employment, they are seldom an adequate substitute for current, specific comment about the person's appropriateness for the position being filled at this time.

In pursuing references, the employing library should be clear in what kinds of information or comment will be most helpful, perhaps providing a brief questionnaire to be completed as well as space for a personal statement on the part of the reference. Every reference needs to be read and interpreted thoughtfully, and some may require follow-up conversation or correspondence.

APPOINTMENTS

Once the decision has been made by the library that an applicant is the person desired for the position, the first person to be notified should be the applicant. If, at that time, the applicant asks for further information or for time to consider the offer, a firm deadline should be set for the response. While some other applicants considered for the same position might at that time be informed that they have not been chosen, it is reasonable to wait for firm acceptance in writing before letting the next one or two candidates know of the decision. If it is necessary to select the second or third choice for the position, it is just as well to be able to leave the impression that they were top choices. Speed and fairness are important at this time. Applicants are sometimes disappointed when a terse letter informs them they have not received the position they wanted, but there is no point in entering into lengthy correspondence about their strengths and weaknesses as contrasted with those of the successful applicant. If one of the people who wanted the job calls or writes to ask for further reasons why it was given to someone else, the administrator responsible for the selection should reply without making comparisons among candidates, but simply noting what factors were considered by those making the decision in which the applicant was not as strong as needed for the position.

Inquiries about not being selected can become serious if suits or legal action are threatened on grounds of unfair selection. For that reason, it is essential to keep full, accurate records of all applications, notes from interviews, evaluations (especially if more than one person participated in interviewing candidates), and all related correspondence.

The fact remains, however, that even if two candidates seem to the person selecting for the position to be neck and neck with many similarities, there is only one job to be filled. This is sometimes difficult for newcomers to the job market to comprehend. Having gone through educational programs where 10 people could get 100% on a test if that was the score they earned, they find it hard to accept rejection if their own credentials appear to be equivalent to those of the person selected. For this reason, the noncommittal attitude recommended at hte time of the interview is important, as is thorough sharing of evaluations among the people who may have participated in the interview process on the part of the library.

PERFORMANCE EVALUATIONS

Once an employee has been accepted for a position at the public library, available opportunities and corresponding responsibilities have only begun to be explored. The employee has the right to expect a regular program of evaluation of performance. The initial evaluation should be after the employee has had time for orientation to the job and for performing on a regular enough basis that some judgment of quality can be made, but the evaluation should also be early enough in the employee's work that undesirable behaviors can be identified and corrections recommended.

The employee's special strengths and weaknesses should be reviewed by the immediate supervisor, with comments about areas where further training or work experience may be helpful. Some numerical ratings on such characteristics as attitude toward work, quantity of work, quality of work, attendance and promptness, and potential are useful to give the employee specific information about relative quality as compared with other staff members, but the most significant part of the evaluation may be the written comments of the supervisor and the discussion that occurs during the interview.

Although supervisors may feel that they frequently comment on the work of the employees in their area of responsibility, the formality of a performance evaluation review is important for the individuals concerned as well as for the library. It should be no more threatening than a review of one's assets in other areas, such as a medical check-up or an inventory of household assets. In order for the evaluation to be as valid as possible, the supervisor should prepare the written statement and numerical scores and forward these either to the next level of supervisor or to the administrator responsible for personnel. The purpose here is to have a review that will ensure, to the extent possible, across-the-board fairness and validity in applying standards of measurement of performance. Also, by reviewing the performance evaluations of others, the higher-level supervisor gets a sense of what different supervisors see as significant and also gets information useful in evaluating the supervisory skills of those supervisors.

After this review, the supervisor performing the evaluation should schedule a conference with the individual to be evaluated. Time should be as long as required for good communication, perhaps varying according to individuals, but scheduled at stress-free times when interruptions by telephone or other business are minimal or nonexistent. This interview should allow the employee to question comments made by the supervisor and, especially where negative comments have been made, the supervisor should be prepared to substantiate comments by actual examples.

Evaluations of performance can provide the opportunity for supervisors to learn from employees what changes in work assignment, procedures, or other features of the job might be helpful in improving performance. The goals of the library and of the specific job being performed should be reviewed if necessary for clarification, and the individual may also be encouraged to identify chosen career goals and the place of this job in the achievement of those goals.

TRANSFERS

Policies and procedures concerning transfers within one department or among other departments of the library should be clearly understood and fairly observed. Tempting though it may be to set limits on how long a person should stay with a first job, it is not fair to enforce that requirement on the part of the employee while the library retains the right to transfer people when their skills are more needed in another part of the library. On the other hand, the employee who accepts a position that is open because of special requirements for it—for example, the need for a clerk on a bookmobile to work an unusual schedule or to report for work at different locations—should realize that the appointment was probably based on the individual's ability and willingness to perform that position, and should not spend the first months at work in efforts to get another assignment.

A statement of employment conditions should be presented to all persons at the time of appointment and signed by the employee and the personnel administrator. This should include recognition of the fact that transfers are possible, perhaps even likely, and that they may be initiated by the library administration as well as by the individual. Also included might be references to the fact that occasional or emergency shortages of personnel might at times require the employee to substitute for a short time in another part of the library, and that library public service may require scheduling for evening hours, weekends, or even for customary holidays.

The process to be followed in announcing transfer opportunities should allow all employees equal access to the information on a timely basis. The most difficult problems here are the tendency of the personnel administrator to be pressed to fill a position as rapidly as possible, the initiative of some staff members to find out about and request transfers before information about them has reached everyone, and the difficulty of envisioning how the known capacities of a staff member can be evaluated in a position that may be at the same level but which requires different skills. It is sometimes easier for the supervisor interviewing people for a position to evaluate the strengths of a person who has not been previously employed by the library as superior to those of a person who has worked for other supervisors. Special care needs to be taken to be fair in instances like this.

Transfers can provide new stimulus to employees and enhance their self-images as well as their value to the library. Sometimes transfers can correct problems that have developed. For example, when a position opens nearer the home of an employee who has had to struggle with a long commute to the place of work, that person may benefit from the transfer and, at the same time, the library benefits from retaining the person and having a grateful employee who will be more prompt and perhaps even more available to assist in emergency situations by reporting on short notice.

Transfers should not be attempted in order to correct serious personnel problems without having them recorded. The instance noted above is one where a transfer can have double benefits. There are also times when personal conflicts or strong differences about the appropriate role of the library may make the transfer of a person from one supervisor to another desirable, but, in these instances, the reason for the transfer should be recorded. Too often an individual becomes a kind of flying Dutchman of discontent and poor performance, moving from one part of the library to another, perhaps even back again to earlier assignments, because no one supervisor early in the game noted real problems of attitude or performance. Time goes by, and the individual becomes a long-term employee difficult or impossible for the library to terminate, and the record of transfers is all that suggests the difficulty because for a few people, early in the person's employment, it was easier to transfer than to discipline or to train or terminate.

PROMOTION

Promotional opportunities should be announced throughout the library as promptly and as regularly as possible. Brief announcements of individual promotional opportunities may increase the pool of applicants and call to the attention of those who are not eligible or interested that promotional opportunities do exist, and that current employees are encouraged to seek them. As noted in the section about recruitment, there may be negative repercussions if numerous promotional opportunities are announced, giving employees the impression that all upper-level personnel are moving out of the library. For that reason, it may be a good idea to include in the announcement a brief statement about the reason for the opening, such as the incumbent's move out of the city, retirement, etc.

Ideally, the lines of communication among persons interested in promotion, their supervisors, and the administrator responsible for personnel should be clear enough that, when a position is open, the supervisor and the administrator have some idea of who within the library is qualified, interested, and ready for such appointment. Some individuals may need to be encouraged to apply, and, if they are, it should be clearly stated that they may not be selected for the position, but that their qualifications are such that they are encouraged to consider the possibility of applying. Applicants for promotion who come from within the library probably deserve some special consideration in the promotion process. If applications are numerous, not all applicants may be interviewed, but all of those from within the library should have that opportunity. If an individual is applying for a position in another part of the library, it should be feasible to consider the possibility of promotion without requiring that the person's supervisor be informed. Later, if the promotion is likely to occur, the individual should be given the opportunity to inform the current supervisor of his interest and the likelihood of his being promoted at that time.

There are times when some positions are underfilled. For example, a senior employee at a higher level may leave and be replaced, either for lack of funds or as part of a major austerity plan, by a person at a lower level. When the opportunity comes to raise the level of that position again, the incumbent who has done an effective job should be given the promotion, and, throughout the intervening period, the library should make clear its plan for this equitable arrangement when it can be accomplished. Since a promotional opportunity of this kind is not announced, there may be some negative comments from employees about inconsistency, but if the arrangements are open and clear, such comments can be fairly refuted.

LEAVE OF ABSENCE/REINSTATEMENT

Permanent employees often have the prerogative of requesting and being granted leaves of absence. These are periods of set time when they are on leave without pay. Information about these leaves should be available in employee handbooks or separate memoranda so that employees may consider their options in seeking them.

Reasons for leaves of absence may include military service, education, illness, extended travel, and family responsibilities, to name a few. It is often customary to limit the employee from working in some other position during a leave of absence, but there may be reasonable exceptions to that policy. The value of this benefit lies in assuring the employee that a position, not necessarily the one from which leave was taken, will be available on some priority basis upon the employee's return. The governmental unit of which the public library is a part may have policies and procedures concerning these leaves about which the library should inform employees. For example, people who take leave for military service often have the highest priority for reappointment upon their return.

Employees are well advised to request the longest period of time they may need, especially if they have the option of returning in a shorter period of time in case their commitments or plans should change. The risks and the benefits of leaves of absence should be clear to them. The risks include the fact that the same position from which they took leave may be unlikely to be open upon their return, and there may be delay in reappointing them if all positions at their former level are filled at the time they are available again. The benefits include the option of retaining a position at a level above the beginning level if that is what they presently hold, but it is frequent practice that, upon return, the employee reverts to the lowest salary level for the position held, that is, being reinstated at the first step of the salary level for that grade of position, rather than at the level held at the time leave was granted. Another benefit may be the opportunity of continuing in the pension system, the insurance plan, and other staff benefits, although increased payments may be required for these plans if the individual is to continue in them during the period of leave.

Because employees may be under special stress at the time of asking for leaves of absence, it is essential that the terms of the leave—amount of time, process for requesting an extension, protocol for making the request, possibility of delay in reappointment, for example—be clearly stated in writing and signatures affixed both by the representative for the library and the employee. The administrator responsible for personnel should also maintain a file that records who is on leave and what their status is. If the limit of the leave is about to be reached, the administrator may send a reminder to the employee that an extension should be requested or the employee should plan to return to work. Also, it is clear that not all requests for leave can be granted. If the prospect of reappointment is severely curtailed by the number of employees taking advantage of this prerogative, some limitation may need to be placed on the numbers to whom leaves are granted. It is important to keep in mind that the granting of a leave of absence is a privilege, and that the purpose of these leaves is to continue the association of good employees with the library, not simply to stimulate them to be away for some periods of time and to return at their leisure and convenience.

When leaves of absence exceed more than a month or so, it should be taken for granted that the position vacated by the person on leave should be filled by someone else. In most instances, such an appointment should be permanent if the newly appointed person meets the criteria for the position, and it should be clearly understood, as noted above, that the person returning from leave is entitled only to a comparable position, not to the same position from which leave was taken.

RETIREMENTS, RESIGNATIONS, AND TERMINATIONS

Many reasons can cause an employee to leave a position in a public library. Retirements and resignations are usually voluntary, although in some instances, employees may be counseled to consider them, for instance, when continuing ill health has affected their performance or when financial benefits for them may be better realized by seeking retirement than by continuing to work. Retirements for physical disability may follow leaves of absence, and it should be possible for employees to go from a leave into retirement without returning to work. Since all employees may not have been at the library long enough to participate in a pension program or to receive any pension benefits, it should be noted that those who leave without such benefits are resigning rather than retiring, and the terms should not be confused. The administrator responsible for personnel should provide to all employees at time of initial employment the information needed about retirement benefits, and periodic review of those benefits on an individual or group basis should also be available.

Some employees prefer to plan for their retirements without extensive discussion with others about the date or such circumstances as their age or physical condition. For them, frequent group couneling opportunities may provide the information they need about how to start their retirements without violating the privacy they wish to maintain. However, in order to maintain good morale and staffing patterns, the library must receive information about forthcoming retirements on a timely basis. The required length of time before retirement that the individual should give notice should be clearly stated, and information about the procedure for initiating retirement should be generally available.

The procedure for resignations should also be clear, with employees informed as soon as they begin work about the length of notice required when submitting resignations and about what effect their resignation may have on the amount of vacation time available to them, the payment of their library-related insurance premiums, etc. Employees probably should be encouraged to consult with the administrator responsible for personnel when they are planning to resign so that the paper work associated with resignation is prepared appropriately. For example, the employee may inform the library of a last day of work and become confused about the amount of vacation time, the scheduling of days off, or other factors that affect what the last paid day of employment may be.

Often, employees may investigate the possibility of resigning and not follow through on their plans. The administrator responsible for personnel may feel some frustration at hearing frequent comments about forthcoming resignations that do not materialize, and good planning for staff deployment may be adversely affected if resignations are anticipated but not made formal. At this point, however, the employee's right to determine the circumstances of resignation is important to maintain.

Counseling and interviewing for persons planning to resign should include investigation of other options. If changes of assignment or potential for promotion can honestly be forecast and used to continue the employment of a valued person, these should be explored and recommended. If the person is intending to move to another part of the country, but does not have definite plans for employment there, the administrator may wish to suggest a leave of absence rather than a resignation if that would make it possible for the individual to return if the relocation does not prove to be satisfactory. The administrator may also assist in the individual's job search, an effort that can have many positive effects.

In any case, an exit interview conducted sufficiently in advance of the employee's leaving the library can be productive in several respects. Problems the employee has encountered, but has not reported previously, may come to light in this kind of interview, and they can often be corrected for the future. Communication may be more effective at this time than at many others to get insight into what other employees see as problems with the library, and this is also the last opportunity for the administrator to respond to such concerns with some of the background or rationale for decisions, which may have been inadequately conveyed in the past.

The responsibility for terminating an individual's employment is one of the most onerous, painful ones that face an administrator. When termination is for cause, that is, required because of the employee's inability or unwillingness to perform the job satisfactorily or because of theft, gross misbehavior, or other major personal problems, there should, in most instances, be a record of earlier efforts to correct the problem or to limit its seriousness through discipline, example, and training. Since termination is the harshest punishment an individual employee can receive, it should be based on sound evidence of wrongdoing when that is the reason, and it should be decided as promptly as possible, with the employee informed of the decision while the link between the decision and the cause for termination is clear.

There are other instances in which the library must terminate the services of an employee. When a major shift of emphasis in the role and goals of the library occurs, some employees may need to be terminated even when their work has been satisfactory. More frequently, this may be the case when budget cuts or reallocation of available funds require a reduction in personnel. These terminations can be painful for the responsible administrator as well as for the affected employee, but it is important for them to be handled in a humane, businesslike, unsentimental way. The administrator may make exceptional efforts to assist employees in this instance to find appropriate employment, but false hope about the possibility of reemployment should be carefully avoided. Such attitudes hurt, rather than help, the employee.

A layoff policy should be prepared by the personnel administrator with advice and assistance from relevant staff members, and it should be presented to the public library's board for approval as formal policy. Like a policy on selection of materials, this policy should be prepared and in place before there is need for it or controversy about individual applications of it. The policy should state clearly the criteria to be followed in the event of the need for layoffs of personnel. Seniority, with distinctions between seniority in grade and seniority in library employment, may be one criterion. Marginal performance evaluations may be cause for some terminations in times of austerity, even though the evaluations would not otherwise justify termination. Employees in programs considered less than essential might also be candidates for layoff, but it should be noted that the criteria suggested here need to be combined. There may be valued senior employees in marginal programs, for example, and the policy should allow for them to be moved into positions to be maintained, with the employees in those positions placed in the category of those to be laid off if such action is required.

In all instances when an employee leaves the public library, there should be a checklist of information maintained. Keys may need to be returned, information should be obtained about appropriate forwarding address for final paychecks and income tax reports, and review of library property for which the individual was responsible should be carefully made. While supervisors may take some of the responsibility for this, the administrator responsible for personnel should be aware of the need for these measures and should, if necessary, hold the final paycheck until the employee's responsibilities to the library have been fulfilled.

TRAINING

The training that a library customarily provides in order to enable its employees to perform their work within the library is diverse. Initially, orientation sessions that introduce groups of employees to the functions and goals of the library, preferably providing an opportunity to get the views of major administrative personnel, should be scheduled on a regular basis so that new employees get this orientation within their first weeks of work.

Inservice programs, usually extending over a period of time, may include introduction to some specific job-related skills, such as public speaking, circulation management, data processing, or other tasks that the library requires employees to master. While there are benefits to the library employee in acquiring these skills, the major purpose of the programs is to improve the operation of the library, and, for that reason, attendance and active participation may be required, no fees charged for the training, and no academic credit received for the program.

Because they are less formal in nature, the guidance and supervision given to employees are not always recognized as vital parts of training, but they are in fact. Immediate supervisors may administer most of this aspect of training, and some informal records should be kept of what is taught in the course of the employee's performance of a job. This record is useful in determining whether the employee is, in fact, ready to accept further responsibility and to acquire additional skills, and it may also need to be kept for reference about the length of time it takes an employee to acquire a skill or to develop full competence and speed in performance. For example, if a staff member at the circulation desk is to be expected to be in complete charge of the circulation procedure for a day or an evening, it should be possible to verify that all aspects of circulation and registration of borrowers have been carefully explained and learned by the staff member.

In all of these training activities, there should be a two-way evaluation. If training is required and if staff members go to training sessions on library time, their presence should be noted; if a skill is being learned or information about a new procedure is being provided, they should have some simple test on their new competence. They may also have the responsibility of reporting on their training to others and perhaps of teaching others within their unit or department what they have had the opportunity to learn.

The second part of the two-way evaluation is of special concern to the administrator responsible for personnel. This is the employee's opportunity and responsibility to evaluate the format and content of the training received. While there are incidental benefits to this—improvement of morale by providing for response by employees, provision of the opportunity for individuals to comment, and reminding the person giving the training of the need for good quality of performance—the major value should be the assistance that such evaluations give in the planning of future training. If sessions are too long, rooms too warm, directions unclear, etc., these are matters which can and should be corrected—but they need to be known. By the same token, it is highly desirable that these evaluations should be received as soon as possible after the training experience, while memories and criticisms are fresh.

The timing of other aspects of training is always important. When training is required to introduce a new procedure or a new technology, it should be provided as near as possible to the time that the procedure or technology will be in use. Prompt utilization of new skills is a fairly sure way to retain them, but some further review of the procedures or skills may be desirable after they have been utilized for a time.

STAFF DEVELOPMENT

Just as training has been interpreted here to refer to the acquisition of skills needed by library employees to function effectively in their job assignments, staff development is the term used for the many aspects of continuing education that provide more benefits to the employee in terms of continuing career development than to the library in terms of accomplishment of its goals. The line between training and staff development is sometimes a thin one, and it is certainly true that the library often benefits from an employee's continuing an educational program and that the employee may enhance his career opportunities by taking the library's training.

Workshops may be conducted by library-related organizations or by other job-related groups such as secretarial groups or by institutions of higher education. These are usually one-time opportunities, with emphasis on the development of a single skill or introduction of concerns about a single aspect of library service, such as service to the deaf. It is difficult to assess the quality of such workshops in advance of their being available, but the library's personnel function should include announcing the availability of such opportunities, advising individuals who are interested in attending them, and noting the ways in which such workshops may intersect with the library's own program of training.

Participation in job-related organizations is important for the well-being of the individual as well as for the improvement of the library. Clear policies and procedures should exist about the extent of the library's support of such activities, and these should be prepared with concern for the new employee anxious to become active as well as for the veteran who may already have given generously of time and energy but who wishes to be able to continue to be active. It should be understood that some of the time, money, and responsibility required for these activities should come from the individual, with such support by the library as is feasible.

Participation in formal academic courses may be encouraged by the public library in several ways. Time may be allowed so that employees can attend classes, or schedules adjusted to encourage their continuing their education on their own time. Provisions for reimbursement of tuition can be one of the greatest encouragements of all, but it can also be a major investment. Some concern may be exerted here to review the relevance of the course work to the employee's present job or future job prospects within the library, but it should be kept in mind that academic challenge and mental stimulation can have positive effects on staff members whether or not the content of the courses they choose is closely related to their work in the library.

When the public library needs people with special skills, such as the ability to speak a foreign language, it may make as much sense to provide the time, opportunity, and money for several people to acquire these skills as to search to recruit personnel who already possess the skills. In these instances, the academic study clearly benefits the person on the job as well as the library, but it may make more sense for the courss to be taken as part of a formal academic program than within the setting of the library's training program.

In all aspects of training and continuing education, library administrators should be alert to ways of combining their efforts to provide training and continuing education for their staff with the efforts of other groups within the same governmental unit or with nearby libraries. There are often benefits to be obtained by having a larger group participate in educational programs and in having a more diverse group of participants.

Participation in job-related organizations is likely to lead to interest in attending conferences, requests to receive support for travel, and use of library time for committee work and other activities associated with participation in such associations. Guidelines for making such requests should be clear, and fair administration requires open communication of the criteria to be used in making decisions about which and how many staff members attend conferences, receive travel reimbursement, and on what basis library time may be used for association-related activities.

There is probably no better encouragement to staff than the model of supervisors who participate in professional organizations and who strike a balance between the contribution of their own time and money to such activities and the requests they make of the library. Staff may occasionally need to be reminded that the provision of their time, when it might otherwise be devoted specifically to the library, is an investment by the library also, and that although travel funds may be limited or nonexistent, the allowance of time to attend conferences is an expense that can best be realized when the hours of staff time are translated into dollar figures.

In this and in other areas, the administrator responsible for personnel may find that the effort to support staff activities requires considerable persuasive power to receive support from the library's board of trustees, the political administrators in whose areas the library operates, and the public at large. The most cogent reasons for such support are probably the benefits the library receives from this kind of activity. First, the activity is a means of continuing education for staff members, and it is a factor in good staff morale. More than that, however, may be the prestige the library derives from effective contributions of its staff members, a value that, in turn, stimulates the interest of recruits in the library and extends its public awareness program throughout the library profession and, when the same or similar benefits are permitted to other specialists within the library, throughout other professions or specializations also.

Just as systematic as the means by which employees seek and receive approvals to attend conferences or otherwise participate in job-related organizations should be the means by which they report. Since not all employees may participate in these activities, it is important that those who do should share with others what they have learned and observed and what they have concluded as a result of it. Oral presentations to the staff as a whole, written reports for the staff newsletter, sharing of materials (posters, exhibitors' catalogs, cassettes of speeches, to name a few) with others in the library are good ways to extend the value of such opportunities.

It is important for the personnel administrator and other supervisors to keep in mind that there are likely to be some staff members who will be constantly alert and eager to take advantage of all kinds of continuing education opportunities, while some may seldom consider such possibilities. When the benefits of continuing education are not widely sought and used, the positive morale factors can be diminished or even become negative as it appears to staff members that the benefits go only to the few. It is a responsibility of administration to stimulate others to request participation and to review periodically how funds and time allocations have been made to ensure fairness and the best results for the library.

EMPLOYEE COUNSELING

The occasions when employees need to seek professional counseling are usually times of stress for them, when suggestions about the availability of such assistance may be perceived as intrusive and when resentment or anger, rather than appreciation, may be the response. This is as true when the counseling concerns a member of the staff member's family as when it concerns the staff member. For these reasons, it is important that information about the availability of counseling be provided to all employees, and that supervisors be encouraged to have materials about these opportunities handy for individual reference and perhaps occasionally invite to staff meetings speakers who will inform staff about such programs.

Administrators and supervisors frequently possess some of the characteristics of professional counselors, but they should be very wary of attempting to provide professional counseling themselves. One reason that specializations in counseling have developed is that it is extremely difficult for one person to be knowledgeable about various kinds of counseling. The best service that a supervisor or personnel administrator can offer to an employee in need of counseling is reference to a well-qualified counselor.

Typical needs for counseling include alcoholism within the family or on the part of the staff member, career guidance, psychological adjustment, drug abuse, stress, and persistent delinquency. Often, the governmental unit within which the library operates may offer programs for all employees at reduced cost or free. This kind of information should be generously shared with staff members. Where such programs do not exist, the administrator responsible for personnel should ask about the possibility of making them available to staff members on a regular basis.

Emphasis on preventive health care has a corollary here. Counseling is not an activity to be recommended only in crises. It can help to prevent major problems and to maintain the health and perspective of individuals who may not even be aware of the benefits such services can offer.

There may be times when individual supervisors or colleagues of a staff member who seems to require counseling will consult with the personnel administrator about how to encourage the employee to get the necessary help. The more personally this suggestion can be made, the better, in most instances. Supervisors may be reluctant to broach the subject to those whom they supervise, but the personnel administrator may strengthen their resolve by seeing that they have current information to share and by encouraging them to be in touch with a counseling service even before discussing the problem with the employee, especially if free service is available. This communication may alleviate the anxiety of the staff member in need of counseling, and it can certainly mean that the counselor with whom the staff member may or may not communicate is already aware of the problem and prepared to respond.

There are occasions when, in order to continue their work in a productive fashion, staff members may be required to seek counseling. These occur when continued aberrant behavior on the job, extended periods of depression that affect one's work, or clear evidence of alcoholism or drug abuse have had such negative effects that the staff member's job performance is seriously affected. While the individual supervisor may, at these times, advise the staff member that counseling is required if his employment is to be continued, the support of the personnel administrator may be very important to the supervisor making this requirement. If the recommendation is tied to continued employment, a record should be kept of the date and circumstances in which the requirement was made, and the library may further require the staff member to present evidence of participation in counseling sessions.

Counseling is not always successful in correcting a staff member's problems. Painful though it may be, when work performance is so poor that the staff member's employment would be terminated if the cause were something other than this personal problem, then the staff member's employment should be terminated in this instance as well.

RECORD KEEPING

Frequently in the preceding sections, there have been references to the keeping of records. Good record management is an important aspect of good personnel management. Some records, such as personnel files, OSHA reports, progress statements on recruitment and hiring, records of promotions and transfers, and reports of participation in continuing education opportunities, are well known and generally maintained. Others, including records of references, interviews, and information needed to provide personnel assistance, such as counseling resources or continuing education opportunities, are not always retained exclusively in the office of the administrator responsible for personnel, but they may at times be essential for good personnel management.

Some recent legislation and litigation have had major impact on the maintenance of personnel records. Every staff member has the right to review the file pertaining to his recruitment and his period of employment. Many problems can be averted if, as items are added to the individual's file, the filer notes whether a copy has already gone to the individual staff member. Provision of such a copy on a prompt systematic basis may avert some problems. This should apply to performance evaluations, commendations from the public, records of attendance or completion of continuing education programs, as well as to memoranda or letters relating to promotion, transfer, and other standard personnel actions.

One problem in record keeping is the need to balance the right of individuals making personnel decisions to state reasons why they are not recommending promotion or why they are applying discipline or reporting unsatisfactory work performance with the right of the persons affected by those decisions to have full access to the files relating to their work. One solution to this is the one followed in some placement services, in which individuals requesting references from others indicate they have waived their right to read what is written about them. Many users of such files place more credence in statements that they know have not been screened by the individual requesting the reference. Federal and state laws and the policies of the governmental unit in which the public library is located should be carefully read and observed in these matters of privacy and access.

The organization of personnel files should make it possible to: review the employment pattern of any single individual on the staff from recruitment throughout the period of employment, including information about how to communicate with the person after leaving the library; find what the patterns of filling positions have been; enumerate and classify the varieties of personnel actions carried out within set periods of time, such as a month or a year; record the utilization of such opportunities as continuing education and travel on the part of the staff.

There should be clear guidelines available to all staff members with criteria for the kinds of materials that must or should appropriately be added to individual personnel files. In some instances, some compromise may be desirable. For example, if commendations from the public are regularly added to such files, it may be necessary to limit the bulk if one or two staff members receive bundles of material from 20 to 30 members of the public at a time. Refutation of negative comments should be carefully fiied so they are with the comments to which they pertain. Extreme care must be exercised to keep individuals' files separate in spite of similarities of names, dates of appointment, etc. It is usually a good idea to keep files of all current employees in one alphabet, those of potential employees and former employees in two other alphabets. Where space is a problem, files of former employees may need to be weeded of all but the most essential information and stored in a separate area. The confidentiality of these files requires excellence and promptness in maintenance, secure construction of the file cabinets in which they are housed, and concern for good conservation of the papers placed in the files.

Government regulatory agencies, state library agencies, and other agencies at any level of government may make demands or requests for information that require extensive review of massive files unless some notations are made as personnel files are developed. Information, for example, about the numbers of different ethnic groups who were interviewed for a particular position may be requested some time after the position was filled, so that there is value in anticipating such inquiries to the degree possible and noting the information as it is acquired.

There are constraints placed by government regulations on the kinds of information that may be requested or acquired at the time that individuals are recruited for positions, but that same information may later be required about current staff members by the same agency or another one. It may be useful to require employees to complete information cards after their appointment, in which sex, age, ethnic or racial background, and other characteristics are noted. It is also worth the library's while to require that employees be photographed and small photographs be added to their files. These photographs can help to identify employees in case of emergency and may also be useful when several employees are being considered for the same position or for promotion or transfer, and the supervisor concerned wants to be sure of the identity of staff members.

One of the most difficult things to retrieve from personnel files is information about skills possessed by individuals, such as proficiency in foreign languages, ability to play musical instruments, knowledge of keypunching, etc. In the present state of the art, it is often the humane administrator of personnel or the supervisor alert to the special background of staff members who may retrieve that information from memory. The promise of automated personnel files in the future suggests that this kind of information may indeed be readily retrievable. As these systems become available, it is essential that knowledgeable personnel be involved in their development so that the fullest information is recorded and so that retrieval is as efficient and complete as possible.

III
Communication

In many ways, personnel administration can be viewed as a system of communication between the library administration and employees. Several aspects of personnel work rely on specific communication formats and structures. Collective bargaining is a mechanism for management and employees to negotiate the terms and conditions of employment. Grievance procedures provide a vehicle for management to resolve employee complaints. Interviewing is a form of communication that requires certain techniques and is used for several important personnel management activities. Documentation, or record keeping, is a primary function of personnel administration that ensures an accurate and accessible record of employees' work history. Memoranda, forms, meetings, and staff newsletters are methods of communication that convey information in unique formats and styles for specific purposes and audiences.

COLLECTIVE BARGAINING

Collective bargaining is a formal process in which the terms and conditions of employment are negotiated between employees and the library administration. It is a decision-making process that puts the ability to determine such issues as wages, hours, and benefits into the hands of both the administration and the employees. In this sense, it is a process of communicating and negotiating positions with very important consequences. Before the actual negotiations begin, or soon into such talks, several important issues must be resolved. Who will be represented in the union's bargaining units? Who will represent the library administration? How will impasses in the negotiations be resolved? The negotiations themselves consist of a series of proposals and counterproposals that are considered by both sides until compromise or some form of arbitration results in a contract.

The first issue that the library administration must get resolved, either before or at the beginning of the negotiations, is the number and kinds of employees that will be represented by the union. There are two important points to this issue. First, the bargaining units should represent the greatest number of employees possible so that the library can minimize the number of costly negotiation proceedings. In the private sector, bargaining units are primarily derived on the basis of commonality of interests and employee wishes. In public libraries this might translate into clerical, maintenance, and professional units. If this be the case, the library might insist on bargaining with all three units at once in order to avoid having the units play off one another to gain better contracts. The second issue concerns employees who are not union members. The benefits of collective bargaining should apply to all employees who could possibly be in the unit. Unions will generally want to force membership by all employees affected by the bargaining. However, many states prohibit mandatory union membership or "union shop." It is important that these issues be resolved first so that the library can minimize the expense of numerous negotiations and, perhaps more importantly, know how many employees will be affected so that the financial implications of union proposals can be accurately measured.

The library's administration must have adequate and unified representation in the bargaining process. This will ensure that the authority to make commitments is represented along with the management staff who can best judge the impact of union demands on the operaton of the library. Such representation could draw from management personnel, library board members, and officials of parent governmental bodies. Also, the library should seek the advice and services of a lawyer, negotiator, or personnel officer of the encompassing governmental unit in order to have an experienced hand coordinate their side of the negotiations.

The scope of bargainable issues should generally be limited to the terms and conditions of employment. Traditionally, this means wages, hours, benefits, disciplinary procedures, and employment security. However, there are thousands of other issues that have been included in public sector bargaining. The union will want to effect as much change as possible in as many areas as possible to demonstrate its usefulness to its members. Management will want to limit the scope of union influence in order to protect its policy-making discretion. There will be occasions when management may relinquish some authority in trade for union concessions that could reduce the total personnel costs of the contract. For example, the library might agree to curtail summer public service hours, which is a policy issue. In return, the union would agree to productivity concessions that would allow management to reduce staff by having fewer employees take on greater work loads. It is this kind of give and take that is at the heart of the negotiation process.

Within the framework of negotiations, the element of compromise is essential. Both union and management should avoid standing pat on unimportant issues. For that reason, all proposals should be studied closely to determine their actual costs and impacts. Guesswork in these proceedings is counterproductive. However, when an impasse does occur, the private sector allows employees to go out on strike. In the public sector, strikes are very often forbidden by law. Many states have substituted some kind of arbitration procedure for the employees' right to strike. This arbitration can range from fact finding by an objective party who will determine the most reasonable position to binding arbitration that requires both sides to refer disputes to a mediator whose decision must be accepted by both parties. However, these kinds of substitutes have very often failed to prevent strikes. Another unique aspect of public sector collective bargainng has to do with possible conflicts between union contracts and local laws dealing with public employees or civil service regulations. The uncertainty in impasse resolution and conflict with existing laws are just two of the many unique factors that point to the absolute necessity for the library to utilize expert advice. This adviser must be familiar with collective bargaining in the public sector and all local conditions that would affect the environment of local public labor relations.

GRIEVANCES

Grievance procedures are a protocol for employees to communicate their complaints to management and for management to respond to those complaints in a timely and effective manner. Appropriate attention to employee complaints through this kind of mechanism is a cornerstone to good employee relations. Moreover, it gives employees the right to due process even when they are not unionized. The key elements of an effective grievance procedure are clear guidelines as to what is grievable, a structure that allows for appeal to a higher authority, timely response, and a format that is accessible to all employees.

In most organizations complaints are grievable, concerns are not. Complaints are responses to specific incidents in which the employee believes he has been treated unfairly, unequally, or capriciously; or in which some rule, policy, or law has been violated by a supervisor or by management. Generally, salary scales, policies, or terms of a union contract are not considered grievable. In keeping with the limitations on the scope of grievances, and to ensure an objective resolution of a grievance, employees are usually required to document incidents in detail, name witnesses, cite rules violated, and suggest an acceptable resolution.

The structure of the grievance procedure should be such that resolutions can be obtained at the lowest possible level. Appeals should be carried through to higher levels of management. The final arbitration should come from the highest level of authority whose decision is binding and nonappealable. For public libraries, this highest level is usually the library board. At all steps of this appeals hierarchy, time limits should be imposed for a response to the grievance so that the timeliness, hence the effectiveness, of the response is maintained. For many organizations, this time frame is usually one to two weeks for a satisfactory answer.

Employees should be well informed as to what is and is not grievable. In addition, they should have access to the necessary forms, policies, and regulations for filing a grievance. Very often, they are allowed assistance from other employees, lawyers, or a union official for filing the grievance and making presentations at hearings.

It should be emphasized that most grievances are misunderstandings that can be resolved with the immediate supervisor. But the mere fact that the procedure exists gives the employee some recourse, or safety valve, to get a fair hearing on his complaints. Therefore, management should place trust in the grievance procedure it has established. This trust requires that all grievances be handled fairly and quickly. And most importantly, such trust demands that an employee will not suffer reprisals for making use of the grievance mechanism.

INTERVIEWING

At many points of the personnel process, interviewing is important. Hiring, performance evaluation, promotional, and exit interviews are the major ones. Some characteristics apply to all of these. The employee should be asured of the time needed for a useful interview with as few distractions as possible. While settings may sometimes be improvised, as when hiring interviews are conducted in school placement offices or at conferences, they should be businesslike, private, and comfortable.

Preparation for the interviews should include, in most instances, an opportunity for the interviewee to have reviewed any written materials relevant to the interview. An exception to this is the performance evaluation interview, in which the written performance evaluation is presented to the employee as part of the interview. Similarly, the interviewer should be prepared to the extent of having read any information supplied in advance by the interviewee. Questions raised by these materials are often a good way to start the interview.

The hiring interviewer should keep in mind that the purpose of most interviews is not merely to confirm what is already on the record, but to probe the employee to discover whether the strengths he offers to the library are real, while it is the interviewee's task to find out more about the library and its goals, the job under discussion, and to stress the strengths and skills he can offer to it. When hiring or interviewing candidates for promotional opportunities, the interviewer should maintain an interview schedule for each person interviewed, noting the questions essential to be asked of each one and indicating the probing questions that may have been required in some instances. It is sometimes wise to keep the interview moving along a set course even if it is necessary later to return to some points for further clarification or for confirmation of impressions.

The interview should allow for the formalities of introduction and leave-taking without intruding on the times of other candidates who may be scheduled for interviews in the time following. The interviewer should be identified by name and title, and the relationship between the interviewer and the job being discussed should be clear. Especially when applicants are new to the job market, they sometimes have the impression that the person interviewing them will be their supervisor or close colleague, when the interviewer may, in fact, be an administrator at a more remote level.

The results of hiring or promotional interviews should be noted promptly by the interviewer, perhaps using a chart on which the strengths of several applicants can be ranked. It should be possible both for the interviewer and the interviewee to telephone or write or to meet again to clarify any questions that may be unresolved when the interview has been completed. A second interview may also be necessary when a number of people have been interviewed for one position and some of them are being considered more seriously, and there is need to compare them more carefully.

Group interviews, which have been mentioned, may be most desirable when a position is new or when a position has many points of intersection with the work of others throughout the library. Members of the library's board may sometimes participate in these, and so may individuals who will be the peers or the subordinates of the applicant if the appointment is made. The purposes here are to get some consensus on the decision of who the best candidate is, to make the best use of the candidates' time, and to allow participants in the group interview to observe how the applicant interacts with others, listens, and how promptly he may be able to follow a change in the thrust of the questions asked or comments made by those interviewing. For a group interview, the interviewers should review together the information they have received in advance and should prepare individual questions, preferably in their areas of specialization or interest, and review all of these together. A procedure should be clearly stated, and restated in the applicant's presence if necessary, about the procedure for asking questions, allowing time for all concerned to get the information they need to make a recommendation. As in the interview with a single interviewer, there should be time for clear introductions of participants and identification of their concerns with the position being filled. Perhaps more important in the group interview, the interviewee may benefit from having the opportunity to make a brief statement concerning the reason for interest in the position, understanding of what the position involves, and indications of the capacities and potentials the candidate may bring to it.

Exit interviews may range from the euphoric to the violent. Conducted systematically and thoughtfully by the administrator for personnel, they can be the best kinds of evaluations of what is right and what is wrong with the library. The employee who is leaving for a much-desired position or because of a major improvement in his life situation obviously approaches the interview with different feelings from the person leaving because of illness, family problems, or general discontent. Still different is the interview with the individual who has failed to succeed on the job or whose work is being terminated because of cuts in personnel. In all types of exit interviews, however, there is need for two-way exchange of information and interpretation. The personnel administrator should review the employee's personnel file to be sure it is complete and also to see what the nature of work assignments and quality of work have been. If the employee has been marginal in quality, some of the comments he may make about the library or individual supervisors may be of less value than if the work he has performed has always been ranked high. While the notes on the exit interview that are placed in an employee's file should include information about the employee's future plans, address, telephone number, and stated reason for leaving, the long-term value of exit interviews may lie more in what they tell the personnel administrator about the nature of the library, its organization and supervisors, and the attitudes of the employees who make it what it is.

The person conducting the exit interview should verify the employee's work status, noting whether the person intends to seek other work or not and, if so, what kind. Any assistance that can be offered at this time in helping even problem employees find new positions should be stated. A note concerning suggestions, references offered, telephone calls made, or other kinds of assistance provided should be added to the individual's file for future reference and also noted in case there are later inquiries about the library's not providing requisite assistance to employees terminated through no fault of their own.

DOCUMENTATION

Memory and rumor are important communicators of the history of public libraries, and, valuable though they can be, they should not be the substance of personnel decisions and records. Employees and supervisors should be encouraged to document for the record the incidents, developments, and accomplishments that are causes for or are caused by personnel decisions. Sometimes, the records may be kept privately and for short periods of time, as, for example, the notes a supervisor makes about incidents in which a staff member has shown incompetence or rudeness to the public, which are later incorporated into a performance evaluation. Other records may have long-lasting value for the mission of the library, such as recommendations from individual supervisors about how a staffing table should be organized for their areas of responsibilities, or the goals set for one department for a given period of time.

Documentation may be originated outside of the library staff. Commendations of individuals or groups of staff may come from users of the library, and, in most instances, these should be added to the files of the individuals with their knowledge and with a written acknowledgment to the senders. Complaints should also be recorded, but probably not in the file of any individual who may be cited as the cause of them, and they should be investigated and acknowledged. For the personnel administrator, it is important to keep in mind that staff members doing good work may generate complaints, as when an elderly person objects to having the children's librarian preempt some parts of a branch library to teach children how to use the collection, and that staff members doing the wrong thing can generate compliments, as when a staff member at the circulation desk berates a person for late return of library materials to the delight of a taxpayer who is more concerned with seeing the person humiliated or punished than with having the library create a climate of good will and open service. It is important to note trends in complaints and compliments, seeing whether some seasons of the year, some individuals, or some departments yield more comments, and what the reasons for those trends might be.

The format of documentation may be quite varied. Notes written in haste but close to the time of the incident may be better ways to recall the details of an altercation than carefully constructed memoranda written later to record the same events. Actual examples of work may be useful to preserve as part of a record of the quality of a staff member's efforts and achievements. While some administrators may consider writing a log of events, the fact of the matter is that on many occasions a note may be useful if it can be retrieved from a file along the same subject rather than having to be searched for among a lot of disparate notes.

In the matter of personnel changes, there may be several informal comments or inquiries preceding or following any of the library's decisions about promotions, transfers, or other personnel actions. While it may seem to the personnel administrator that memory should suffice for recording such comments, there may be value in recording them more formally. The staff member who asks, apparently on the spur of the moment in the elevator or corridor, about a forthcoming promotional opportunity and receives the answer that no such opportunity exists may be forgotten by the administrator, but if the staff member actually has information about a resignation that is en route to the administrator and later alleges that the administrator discouraged applications, the results in terms of bad feeling and perhaps more serious morale problems are clear. The administrator who regularly records and follows up on even such chance conversations is good for the library, the staff, and personal peace of mind.

Public libraries, attracting as they do staff members who are aware of the value of the written word and the historical record, more often have staff members who overdocument and who believe that the maintenance and sharing of elaborate memoranda about minor problems are valuable activities. In fact, there is no more reason to place trust in written documentation than in oral reports or recollections, especially if the written documentation appears only at times when an individual's word is questioned or when it is offered to substantiate a difference of opinion among staff members. Some balance is needed between the recognition of the value of the written record and the acceptance of conversational comments based on the same facts.

MEMORANDA AND FORMS

The purpose of forms is to make more efficient the communication and retention of information that covers similar items about a number of individuals or that is recorded by a number of different people who may need to be reminded, through the content of the form, of what should be reported. Forms are useful when they make it easier to record necessary information and to organize files so that much similar information can be organized for easy access, but they have little value if they proliferate to the extent that they impede prompt and straightforward communication while the people responsible for such communication search out the appropriate forms or wait to receive them, and then have to struggle to put reports on them that might be stated more clearly in the person's own terms. Tempting though it is for some supervisors and administrators to develop forms that fit their own patterns of providing, gathering, and organizing information, they should be aware of some of the problems forms can cause. In any case, forms should be devised only after a trial basis when their use and filing and content have been tested by a number of users.

Memoranda may be more personal in nature or directed to a group of staff members, the entire board of trustees, or others concerned with the personnel process. Because many such memoranda relating to personnel may need to be prepared within tight constraints of time, it may not always be possible for them to be stated as clearly, even elegantly, as the writer might prefer. Elements of the memoranda should clearly indicate to whom it is directed, from whom it is coming, who else may be receiving copies, the date of its writing and, if it pertains to some recommended or prescribed action, the date it is effective, and the subject. References to actions or memoranda that caused this memorandum to be written should be clear.

Actually, job announcements, performance evaluations, and letters of appointment are all in the category of memoranda, although some may be prepared more like personal letters. When the same information needs to be used in many instances of correspondence, but it is important to make the receiver feel that the letter or memorandum is personal, the use of word processing equipment may be desirable to prepare individual communications without extensive repetitive typing. Especially in matters relating to their work, individuals are extremely sensitive about being recognized as individuals, so special care needs to be taken to have names and addresses complete and accurate and to have the appearance of the communication itself be businesslike, clear, and, to the extent possible, attractive. To have typographical errors in a letter confirming a staff member's termination for careless work may seem funny, and to misspell a person's first name when the individual is leaving library employment after 30 years may also be ludicrous, but both could have serious hurtful effects.

STAFF NEWSLETTERS

In some public libraries, staff newsletters are an administrative tool, while in others, a group such as the staff association takes major responsibility for them, sometimes with administrative support in terms of staff time, supplies, distribution, etc.; in still others, newsletters from the staff association compete with those from administration. Wherever possible, it is a good idea for the newsletter that informs staff about library events, major personnel changes, and similar matters to be prepared cooperatively with staff members contributing to its contents and with the library administration's having access to it for general good communication.

The purpose and protocol of the staff newsletter should be clearly understood by members of the staff and others who receive it. A masthead statement indicating the auspices under which it appears is important, especially if the title of the newsletter is so cute or so general that its origin is not clear. While the brief masthead statement cannot provide it, there should be a statement of policy about the contents of the newsletter, and this should be generally available to staff.

The policy statement should indicate the parameters of the newsletter's contents. Is it to include any personal news of staff members, such as illnesses, weddings, or deaths in the family? Are negative comments about the administration or the efforts of individuals to be permitted? What guidelines might determine the quantity and kinds of public commendations that are included? Are articles to be signed? How is final authority for what is to be included determined? These are some of the questions to which those determining the scope and content of the newsletter need to address themselves.

Public library administrators contemplating the initiation of a staff newsletter or considering the revamping of an existing one would do well to request sample issues of newsletters from public libraries of comparable sizes and select from them ideas they wish to include or exclude. If there is question about a medium-sized or large library's including announcements of events of personal interest to staff members, such as weddings or births, the *Library of Congress Information Bulletin* serves as a good example of a large library's expression of interest in matters of such importance to staff.

The newsletter may be the appropriate place for staff members to report on travel and educational opportunities that they have had. By-lines should probably be permitted on these and similar articles in order to encourage quality in such reporting, to give credit to those making such efforts, and to permit staff members and other readers who want more information to know the possible source of more details.

While a continuing advisory committee for the newsletter may be too formal for some libraries, it is important that the staff be reminded frequently that the newsletter welcomes and responds to recommendations for improvement or change. Essential for a good newsletter are timely information and regular publication. It is better to start a newsletter with the promise of less frequent appearance and to improve its frequency than to make promises about dates of issue that cannot reasonably be met.

If for any reason an issue is delayed, it is preferable to omit information that has lost its timeliness, and to leave out announcements of opportunities for which the deadlines are past than to publicize outdated material that confuses and frustrates readers.

The staff newsletter may be requested by other agencies, such as neighboring libraries, library schools, or the state library agency. Former staff members and board members, especially those who have retired after long association with the library, may also ask to receive the newsletter. For these possible readers, it is a good idea to have a modest subscription price quoted so that distribution costs can be covered and so that the subscriber will have a sense of the value of the newsletter and the option of continuing the subscription if it is of continued interest.

Within the library, the newsletter should provide both a record of the library's accomplishments and announcements of events to come. It should be available to all staff members, possibly on an individual basis, but certainly with multiple copies for each unit so that each staff member can read the entire issue soon after its arrival and without inconveniencing others who also wish to read it.

Valuable though staff newsletters may be as a means of communication between administration and staff and among the various parts of the library, they cannot take the place of memoranda or other announcements relating to personnel opportunities and decisions. For example, individual jobs should be announced separately when applications are being encouraged, so that staff members can peruse such announcements at their leisure, share them with others who may be interested, etc.

MEETINGS

Public library staff members have two customary complaints about meetings: there are too many or there are too few. There should be clear policies about meetings that are to be held regularly, for example, among specialists in a given area, for staff members in a single unit or department, and for representatives of various administrative areas. If meetings are to occur with some regularity, it is probably better to set a schedule of times and places for them and to distribute that to the staff members concerned than it is to try to schedule one meeting during the course of the preceding one. In this regard, the library's administrators can set a sound pattern for others within the library to follow, by scheduling meetings reasonably and with consideration of the library's patterns of public service and other personnel commitments.

When it is essential to get information to a large number of people simultaneously, when questions or comments are welcomed from those in attendance, and when several points of view are to be presented to staff, meetings are probably the best means of achieving these purposes. Any meeting that can be replaced by a memorandum should be.

While formal agendas may not always be necessary for the people attending the meeting, the purpose and scope of the meeting, the length of time scheduled for it, the general format, and the location should be clearly stated in advance. The person convening the meeting needs to have some idea of how much time should be devoted to different parts of the meeting, and should be capable of moving it along on a reasonable schedule, while still allowing for discussion or questions that may be necessary.

The planning and conduct of meetings are skills to be cultivated, especially by administrators and others who wish to be effective leaders in the public library. Deciding when to have meetings, whom to invite as speakers or presenters, how to decide on the appropriate audience, and how to plan such logistical details as coffee breaks, introductions, summaries, and seating arrangements are important for conveners of meetings to know and to practice. The library administration may wish to set some guidelines about who can and should call and conduct some meetings and who should be invited to them. For example, there is little purpose in having public service staff gather to review the problems in prompt receipt and processing of materials unless representatives from the parts of the library responsible for these services are also invited, indeed urged, to attend and respond.

For purposes of good scheduling, the library should maintain a listing of all meetings scheduled in different parts of the library on a fairly long-range basis—for example, for a year at a time. If this listing is consulted by those scheduling meetings, it is possible to avoid such problems as conflict in trying to attract the same people to different meetings at the same time or requiring public services to be poorly staffed while several staff members attend different meetings.

The library's own meetings for staff are the ones discussed here. Elsewhere, there are comments about attendance at other continuing education programs such as professional association meetings. It is important to keep in mind that the library's own meetings for staff are significant as means of providing information, getting responses from the staff, stimulating the two-way communication required by good personnel management, and building sound morale. Other meetings outside the library may supplement these purposes, but they cannot supplant them.

And, since many staff members may, from time to time, have the responsibility for planning and conducting meetings within the library and elsewhere, good models offered by the administration should result in many diverse and long-lasting benefits.

Appendix

Explanation of List and Chart of Elements of Personnel Forms

Personnel records are among the most valuable resources a library has for purposes of administration, current information, and historical review. They should clearly indicate the career of an individual while in the employ of the library. It makes sense for them to be in formats that are customary in the system, whether these be cards, 8½x11 sheets, or whatever is the commonly used material in the library. As noted elsewhere in this book, consistency of personnel actions requires a good file and clearly presented information.

The following chart and list are intended to serve as reminders of what elements of information need to be included on various personnel forms. These are presented in this fashion in order to emphasize the importance of the information, rather than the format in which it might appear. The list indicates the items to which reference is made in the chart by number. This is not a priority listing, but is arranged simply to make identification easier. References to the items mentioned here as part of the personnel file appear elsewhere in the text. In some libraries, other files may be desirable, and other forms essential. They may be fairly easily developed based on these elements.

CHART OF ELEMENTS OF PERSONNEL FORMS

Forms	1	2	3	4	5	6	7	8	9	10	11	12	13	14	15	16	Other Elements
Application for Position	x	x	x	x	x	x	x	x	x	x	x		x	x			References Level/kind of position sought
Reference for Applicant	x	x	x	x	x	x							x				Address of library, Signature of reference, Evaluative comments
Report of Interview of Applicant	x	x	x			x	x	x									Signature of interviewer Evaluative comments
Statement of Conditions of Appointment	x	x	x	x	x	x										x	Comments re length of appointment, salary and benefits, possible hours of employment and location of first assignment
Request for Leave of Absence	x	x	x	x	x	x	x	x				x	x	x	x		
Application for Retirement	x	x	x	x	x	x	x	x				x	x	x		x	Optional: forwarding address
Resignation	x	x	x	x	x	x	x	x					x	x		x	Optional: forwarding address
Termination	x	x	x	x								x	x		x	x	Optional: forwarding address
Exit Interview Report	x	x	x	x		x						x	x			x	

										Approval signatures of supervisor and personnel administrator
Return of Property	x	x x x	x	x x x	x			x x	
Evaluation of Training	x x x	x		x x x		x			
Request for Continuing Education/Travel	x x x x x	x		x x x		x			x x x

LIST OF ELEMENTS OF PERSONNEL FORMS

1—Name of Library
2—Title of form
3—Date of action or request
4—Effective date for action
5—Time span for action requested
6—Identification of applicant/staff member (name and, optionally, Social Security number or other identification)
7—Home address of applicant/staff member
8—Phone number of applicant/staff member
9—Name, address, and phone number of applicant/staff member's next of kin
10—Educational background
11—Experience background
12—Work location—address and phone number
13—Rationale for request
14—Signature of applicant/staff member
15—Signature of supervisor
16—Signature of personnel administrator

Index